the Bread for Life Diet

the Bread for Life Diet

THE HIGH-ON-CARBS WEIGHT-LOSS PLAN

EASY ✦ EFFECTIVE ✦ 100% NUTRITIOUS

Olga Raz, R.D.

Head of Nutrition and Dietetic Unit, Tel Aviv Sourasky Medical Center
Head of School of Nutrition, Ariel Academic College

with Amir Kessner

STEWART, TABORI & CHANG

New York

ISBN 1-58479-463-1

The text of this book was composed in New Baskerville, Memphis & Interstate.
Edited by Debora Yost
Designed by Galen Smith and Nancy Leonard
Graphic Production by Kim Tyner
Printed in the U.S.A.

Stewart, Tabori & Chang is a subsidiary of

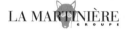

NOTICE: This book is intended as a reference guide, not as a medical guide or manual for self-treatment. If you suspect that you have a medical problem, we urge you to seek medical advice from your health-care provider. Since no two men and no two women are exactly alike, the advice recommended here is not appropriate for everyone. The information is intended to help you make informed decisions about your diet. The recommendations in this book should only be used with the consent and supervision of your primary-care physician or registered dietitian. If you are currently under treatment for any health concern, or are pregnant, get the consent of your doctor before starting this eating program.

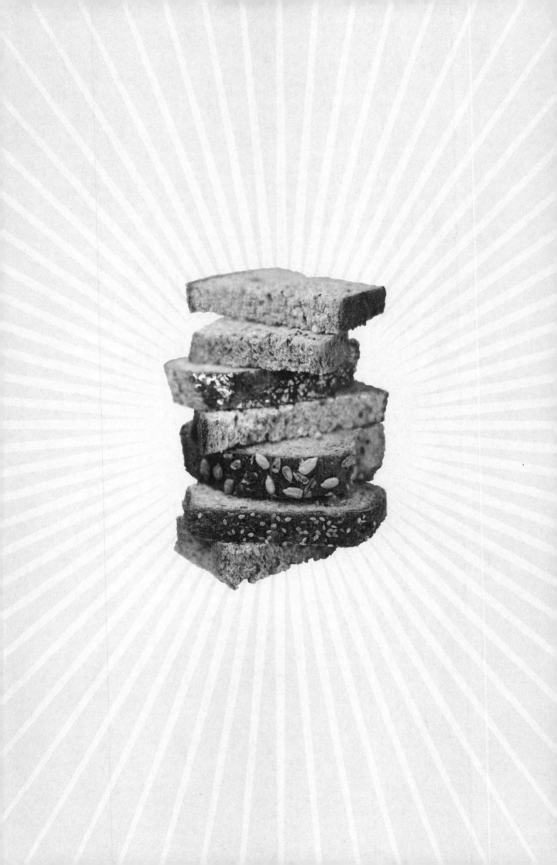

For my daughter,

Nili Raz

✦ ✦ ✦

ACKNOWLEDGMENTS

I would like to thank Professor Ilana Blum, an exceptional individual and scientist, whose broad scientific perspective and boundless energy started me on the road to developing *The Bread for Life Diet*. Approximately 12 years ago, I had the privilege of being a partner in Professor Blum's study of serotonin, which inspired me to develop the diet and eventually write this book.

I would like to thank the entire research team: Dr. Eran Graf, Dr. Yaffa Vered, Dr. Itamar Groskopf, and the dietitian Liora Nassiel (who used part of the joint study in her master's thesis.)

I would also like to extend my profound gratitude to all the clinical dietitians who have done—and continue to do—such wonderful work developing and promoting the "It's All in Your Head" diet program, especially Limor Ben-Haim, Shuli Zemer, Michal Langberg, Liat Hadar, Michal Koltin, Nurit Soroka, and Sharon Maor.

I would like to thank E. A. Tremblay for his help in "Americanizing" the book; Debora Yost, editor at Stewart, Tabori & Chang, whose wise questions and comments helped me very much, and Lisa Andruscavage for her valuable attention to detail.

And last, I would like to thank Aliza Walach, who was the editor of *Eat Bread and Get Slim*, the Hebrew version of this book.

Olga Raz, Tel Aviv, September 2005

CONTENTS

✦ ✦ ✦

Acknowledgments *9*

Chapter 1: *Bread: A New Diet Discovery* *12*

Chapter 2: *Who's Fat, Who's Not* *16*

Chapter 3: *It's All in Your Head* *28*

Chapter 4: *Serotonin & Weight Loss* *41*

Chapter 5: *Insulin & Weight Gain* *52*

Chapter 6: *Who This Diet Can Help* *66*

Chapter 7: *The Bread for Life Diet* *72*

Chapter 8: *Genetics & the Environment* *118*

Chapter 9: *Changing Behaviors: The Six Insights* *126*

Chapter 10: *Energy: It's Still a Balancing Act* *142*

Chapter 11: *Sporty & Thin* *151*

Chapter 12: *An Odd Array of Diets* *161*

Chapter 13: *Secrets of Success* *173*

Chapter 14: *Bread for Life Recipes* *187*

Bibliography *229*

Index *233*

1

Bread: A New Diet Discovery

This book presents a new approach to dieting and weight loss. You'll find it quite different from—and perhaps even contradictory to—most current popular books on the subject. With *The Bread for Life Diet*, you have to eat to lose weight. You are not allowed to be hungry, and you are not restricted to foods high in protein and fat.

In fact, as the title suggests, you are encouraged to eat bread—a lot of bread. You will eat a large number of meals every day, and you will be allowed to eat during the late evening hours, too. The idea is to take the suffering out of dieting and turn the practice of dieting into a natural way of eating that you can do and will want to do for the rest of your life. Hence, the concept of *The Bread for Life Diet*.

The Bread for Life Diet works, and it yields lasting results. This statement is supported by vast clinical experience with thousands of patients. The patients who followed the diet under my guidance lost weight, maintained their new weight, and feel great today. One of the comments I hear repeatedly from people who are following *The Bread for Life Diet* is that they are losing weight but do not even feel as if they are on a diet. This is exactly the goal of the diet and what has made it so successful.

HOW IT ALL BEGAN

I developed *The Bread for Life Diet* in the early 1990s while I was participating in scientific research an the Tel Aviv Sourasky Medical Center, where I am the Head of the Nutrition and Dietetic Unit. In our research, we set out to establish the connection between food and serotonin, one of the brain neurotransmitters influenced by food. Different types of meals were given to healthy volunteers. We found that when people ate a high-protein meal, the serotonin level dropped sharply, and when they ate bread, the serotonin level increased. It is an amazing revelation when you consider that high levels of serotonin provide a feeling of satiety, while low levels can cause hunger and cravings. Our research later was published in medical literature.

The results made me realize that bread, which people fear eating most when dieting, is in fact the most satisfying, the most comforting, and the best satiety-providing food of all. In addition, bread, especially light bread, is relatively low in calories, given its satiety value. A slice of regular bread, feared and missed by so many dieters, has approximately 80 calories, about the same as a container of plain yogurt, and it is so much more satisfying. A slice of light bread, not to be confused with white bread, has about half as many calories, and is almost as satisfying.

With this in mind, I started giving people a diet containing a lot of bread and bread substitutes, together with other foods to make the diet healthful and balanced. That is how *The Bread for Life Diet* was conceived.

In light of the wonderful results people were achieving, I shared the diet with my colleagues, the clinical dietitians at the medical center where I work, and together we developed a weight-loss and maintenance program that we ran in group participation format. We called it the "It's All in Your Head" diet program. My diet groups have been successfully operating since the early 1990s. In 2001, I turned the diet into a book that was published in Israel and Russia (where I was born) under the title *Eat Bread and Get Slim.* The book became a bestseller and has helped thousands more lose weight.

People always seem to react the same when I tell them that they have to eat 10 slices or more of light bread a day. Deeply perplexed and needing clarification, they ask, "You mean 10 slices a *week?*" They are very surprised to learn that 10 slices of bread is the *daily* portion. The bigger surprise, though, comes when they discover how painlessly and efficiently they drop weight while actually eating all that bread!

The average weight loss among healthy people who follow the diet is 10 to 20 pounds in 2 months. Some people lose weight faster or slower, depending on how vigorously they follow the diet. It also depends on their age and how many diets they have been on before, their specific physiology and health problems. Some health problems may impede weight loss and these are covered later in this book. The important thing is that *The Bread for Life Diet* is very diverse (far from being just bread, as you will see) and is much easier to maintain than many other diets. Statistics show that with most diets, only 5 percent of people maintain their weight loss after two years, whereas with *The Bread for Life Diet,* the rate approaches 15 percent.

MANY BENEFITS

During the past few years, I have been researching the health benefits of my diet, with very satisfying results. In addition to weight loss and reduced hip and waist measurements, it significantly reduces the levels of cholesterol, triglycerides, sugar, and insulin in the blood; reduces insulin resistance; and significantly decreases the inflammatory reaction of the body. All these benefits amply demonstrate how healthy the diet is, reaching far beyond the basic aesthetic value of losing weight.

The Bread for Life Diet is based on my research findings and information gleaned from a large number of current scientific studies. I will try to explain, in layman's terms, how your body works, which factors in your body and in the environment slow down weight loss and which speed it up, and what foods will most help you lose weight. Knowledge, after all, gives you power and freedom, and that—along with guidance for real success—is what this book offers.

2

Who's Fat, Who's Not

Is obesity in the eye of the beholder? You may be tempted to think so. Many people believe that they are overweight, even if no one else sees them that way. Try this experiment: Choose some friends or family members of average weight and ask them if, in their own opinion, they think they could stand to lose a few pounds. Odds are that you will get an unhesitating "yes," especially from women, no matter how lean they are.

"You can never be too rich or too thin" has become a motto of our times. Just look at the ideals of beauty our culture holds up for us: pop stars, supermodels, and fitness gurus, to name just a few. We are left believing that there is something wrong with us if we are not pencil thin, or that we have a character flaw if we don't keep calorie consumption down to starvation levels, even with a barrage of advertisements trying to entice us to buy an infinite variety of junk foods. Guess what? We've been scammed.

YOU ARE WHO YOU ARE

The truth is that most of us are unable to be too skinny, no matter how hard we try. We are just not designed to be that way. Each individual accumulates fat at a rate and to a degree different from everyone else. That makes some people naturally thinner than others. Likewise, some people have straight hair and others curly, some have pale skin and others dark, and some are tall while others are short. We may wish we had another person's hair, coloring, or stature, but wishing will not make it so. In the same way, when it comes to body weight, we cannot have the body we admire on someone else. Nature will not allow it.

IS IT PSYCHOLOGY?

We often try to justify obesity with psychological claims such as:
I'm fat because my mother was too cold toward me.
I'm fat because my father was too demanding.
I'm fat because I'm afraid to attract men.
There's no doubt that these claims hold some truth and that they do help explain the development of obesity. However, it is most important to understand that there are fundamental genetic differences among human beings with regard to their ability to store fat. Grasping this concept can help us come to terms with how we are built so we can stop perceiving our shape and measurements as a defect or disability. Only then might we find it easier to lose weight.

So, if we cannot all be "model" slim, how can we know if we are over-weight or just the right size? If it is not the emaciated images presented to us in the media, what is an objective definition of overweight?

In the past, one common practice was to use height as a guide for determining proper weight for males and females. Using this premise, tables were compiled by the Metropolitan Life Insurance Company in 1943, based on the knowledge that obesity is, without a doubt, a risk to one's health. Using these tables to establish an "ideal" weight, however, is pretty absurd. After all, what is "ideal"?

Gradually, it became quite clear that millions of people of similar height are not the same weight and that factors other than height can affect how high the scale goes when you step on it. In 1983, the insurance company improved the tables by factoring in such variables as gender, frame size, age, and physical activity levels. Later, new data were added by the National Health and Nutrition Examination Survey (NHANES) and others. Today, for each defined height, the weights listed take these factors into consideration and the ranges are described in terms of *desirable weight* and *healthy weight.*

FIND YOUR SIZE

Using the tables on pages 19 and 20, you can determine your "optimal" weight, as opposed to the impractical Barbie doll weight you may dream about and torture yourself to achieve through extreme diets. Refer to the table that corresponds to your gender, and locate the weight that corre-sponds to your height and body frame. Add 2 to 3 percent to the listed weight for every 5 years you are over the age of 59.

Note that these tables will give you only a rough estimate of your desirable weight. You should determine the most desirable weight for you in consultation with your primary care physician or clinical dietitian.

DESIRABLE HEIGHT-WEIGHT

(Ages 25 to 59)

MEN				
Wearing indoor clothing weighing 5 pounds and shoes with 1-inch heels.				
Height			Frame	
FEET	INCHES	SMALL	MEDIUM	LARGE
5	2	128-134	131-141	138-150
5	3	130-136	133-143	140-153
5	4	132-138	135-145	142-156
5	5	134-140	137-148	144-160
5	6	136-142	139-151	146-164
5	7	138-145	142-154	149-168
5	8	140-148	145-157	152-172
5	9	142-151	148-160	155-176
5	10	144-154	151-163	158-180
5	11	146-157	154-166	161-184
6	0	149-160	157-170	164-188
6	1	152-164	160-174	168-192
6	2	155-168	164-178	172-197
6	3	158-172	167-182	176-202
6	4	162-176	171-187	181-207

Source: *Modern Nutrition in Health and Disease,* 9th ed. (Lippincott Williams & Wilkins) 1999.

DESIRABLE HEIGHT-WEIGHT

(Ages 25 to 59)

✦ ✦ ✦

WOMEN				
Wearing indoor clothing weighing 3 pounds and shoes with 1-inch heels.				
Height			Frame	
FEET	INCHES	SMALL	MEDIUM	LARGE
4	10	102-111	109-121	118-131
4	11	102-113	111-123	120-134
5	0	104-115	113-126	122-137
5	1	106-118	115-129	125-140
5	2	108-121	118-132	128-143 ~ 135
5	3	111-124	121-135	131-147
5	4	114-127	124-138	134-151
5	5	117-130	127-141	137-155
5	6	120-133	130-144	140-159
5	7	123-136	133-147	143-163
5	8	126-139	136-150	146-167
5	9	129-142	139-153	149-170
5	10	132-145	142-156	152-173
5	11	135-148	145-159	155-176
6	0	138-151	148-162	158-179

Source: *Modern Nutrition in Health and Disease,* 9th ed. (Lippincott Williams & Wilkins) 1999.

WHAT IS BODY MASS INDEX?

Another way of determining the degree to which a person may be overweight is by calculating his or her Body Mass Index (BMI). Due to its simplicity, BMI is used primarily in scientific studies and statistical calculations and therefore follows the metric system.

To compute your BMI, divide your weight, in kilograms, by your height, in meters, and divide that answer by your height, in meters, again. In other words

$$BMI = kgs. \div m. \div m.$$

For those used to the American system, the BMI can be calculated by multiplying your weight, in pounds, by 702, dividing the answer by your height, in inches, and dividing that answer by the height, in inches, again. In other words

$$BMI = 702 \times lbs. \div in. \div in.$$

For example, let's calculate the BMI for a person who is 1.70 meters tall and weighs 83.3 kg. Divide 83.8 by 1.7 and divide it by 1.7 again, yielding 29. Let's use the American system to calculate the BMI for the same example as above—a person who is 5'7" (67 inches) and weighs 185 pounds. Multiply 702 by 185, then divide the answer by 67 and divide it by 67 again, yielding 29.

Interpreting BMI Values

Underweight	Less than 20
Optimal weight	20-25
Moderately overweight	25-30
Obesity	30-40
Severe obesity	40 and above

Optimal BMI Values by Age

Age	Normal BMI Values
19-35	20-25
35-45	21-26
45 and above	22-27

Choose the BMI you want to attain and use it to calculate your corresponding desirable weight. However, do not go too low because it may be a goal that is too hard to achieve. Simply multiply your height squared by the desired BMI value, then divide that answer by 702.

in. x in. x BMI ÷ 702

The same 5'7" (67-inch) person would multiply 67 by 67, then multiply that answer by 25, and divide by 702. The result is 160 pounds, meaning that the person in our example should lose 25 pounds in order to reach the weight with a BMI value of 25. You can choose any BMI value in the normal range, according to your age, to determine your healthy weight.

FACTORS THAT AFFECT WEIGHT

Just as with the height-weight tables, BMI is not a perfect measure in determining if you are overweight. Not only is everyone different but it does not take into account frame size and gender. When figuring out your healthy body weight and desired BMI, there are other factors you must take into consideration.

Gender. There is a natural difference in weight between women and men of the same height. Women normally carry a higher percentage of body fat than men do, and this difference exists even from early childhood. The source of the difference lies in an ancient survival mechanism.

In the distant past, when women's main physiological and biological role was giving birth and they got pregnant frequently, women's bodies stored fat so that when food was scarce, they would still be able to provide nourishment for their fetuses and breastfeed their babies.

Fat is also important for the production of one of the estrogen derivatives necessary for the secretion of other female sex hormones, a fact that links fat tissue to fertility. Women's greater ability to store fat is a characteristic inherent in their genes, and the compulsive war against it can be exhausting and even harmful.

Age. As we grow older, our metabolism slows down and we become less active, so eventually we start to gain weight. Again, this is a kind of ancient survival mechanism. The older a person got, the harder it was to gather food, so nature partly compensated with the ability to store fat. Women, in particular, suffer from age-related weight gain and accumulation of fat, which begins some 10 years before the cessation of menstruation. This is why so many women age 40 and over complain that they are eating the same amounts as they used to but now they are gaining weight. Weight gain after menopause is related to hormonal changes, among other factors. This tendency stops near the age of 75, when many people start losing weight.

Frame size. Body frames are categorized into three sizes: small, medium, and large. Frame size relates mainly to the structure of the skeleton—the larger the skeleton, the higher the optimal weight. To get a rough idea of your frame size, wrap the thumb and middle finger of the hand you write with around the wrist of the hand you do not write with. If your middle finger and thumb overlap, you have a small frame; if your middle finger and thumb just touch, you have a medium frame; and if your middle finger and thumb do not meet, you have a large frame.

Physical activity levels. Regular physical activity helps reduce fat tissue. However, many athletes weigh more than their nonathletic counterparts. Does this mean that those athletes are fatter? Most definitely not. It usually means that they carry more muscle, which is heavier than fat of the same volume.

WHY FAT BUILDS

Every time we lose weight, fat is broken down, but so is muscle. When we regain weight, we accumulate mainly fat. That's why whenever we repeatedly lose and regain weight, we get fatter and fatter: percentage of body fat goes up. A proper diet together with physical activity helps reduce the amount of fat accumulated in fat tissue while minimizing the damage to muscles.

PERCENTAGE OF FAT

Another important index for defining obesity is percentage of body fat. It is excess *fat*, not excess *weight*, that is responsible for putting us at risk for health problems.

If you wish to get an accurate measurement of your body fat, special instruments can be found in hospitals, fitness clubs, private clinics, and so forth. One of the most accurate tests done in hospitals and medical centers is called DEXA (Dual Energy X-ray Absorptiometry), which performs the measurements by using X-ray. Another technique, called bioimpedance, measures the electrical conductivity of body liquids to calculate body fat. The bioimpedance technology has been captured in a special step-on scale, which can usually be found in private clinics and in fitness clubs, though they are available for home use from bed and bath specialty stores and department stores. While less accurate than DEXA, the scale still gives some indication of changes in body fat as a result of diet and exercise. You usually can see the percentage go down after a few weeks.

THE TWO MAIN TYPES OF OBESITY

You may have noticed that people tend to accumulate fat on different areas of their bodies. There are two main types of obesity, which are named based on the location of accumulated fat: abdominal (belly) obesity and thigh (hip) obesity. Abdominal obesity is more common in men and causes what is popularly known as an "apple shape." Thigh obesity is more common in women and causes what is popularly known as a "pear shape." There are, of course, women with apple-shape obesity and men with pear-shape obesity, as well as mixed types.

Apple-shape obesity is characterized by the accumulation of fat in the upper abdominal area, creating the potbelly. Fat cells in this area, which have the ability to expand and grow, are capable of storing huge amounts of fat. In addition to being aesthetically unappealing, this type of obesity is also associated with various health risks. As fat fills the abdominal cavity, it can cover internal organs, such as the heart and the liver. The hearts of people with apple-shape obesity are yellow rather than red, and their livers are yellowish-brown instead of dark red.

Apple-shape obesity is a part of metabolic syndrome, or syndrome X, which is a cluster of several known symptoms that lead to heart disease, such as hyperinsulinemia (excessive insulin in the blood), high blood sugar and triglycerides, diabetes, high blood pressure, and decreased levels of "good" HDL cholesterol. Research shows that abdominal fat is very active in producing various substances, such as cytokines (which add to the risk of cardiovascular disease by inducing sub-clinical inflammation), that can impair normal blood flow and increase the risk of blood clot production. There are other health problems connected with apple-shape obesity, such as cancer, gout, and male and female infertility. When weight loss occurs, the fat cells become smaller and smaller, cytokine levels decrease and so, too, do many health risks.

Incidentally, there are thin men with abdominal obesity, and they have the same health risks. The good news is that treatment of this type of obesity is relatively easy with the proper diet, and weight loss is faster than in pear-shape obesity. Apple-shape obesity in women usually occurs in those who have a hormonal imbalance, such as diabetes, polycystic ovaries or high cortisol levels.

Pear-shape obesity does not usually result in the same health risks that are associated with abdominal obesity. Most of the health-related problems caused by pear-shape obesity are related to carrying excess weight, such as damage to the knees and other parts of the legs. Treatment is more problematic, however, because the number of fat cells in the thighs and buttocks is extremely high, making weight loss more difficult. That's why women who diet often express frustration at the fact that the result is often a thinning of the face, but not of the buttocks. I often try to convince my female patients not to lose too much weight, as I believe the face is more important than the buttocks. I'm still surprised each time I encounter a woman who thinks otherwise.

Determining whether you have apple-shape obesity is very simple: Measure the circumference of your waist. If you are a man with a waist that measures 41 inches or above or a woman with a waist measuring 35 inches or above, it means that you have abdominal obesity, with all of its associated health risks. You should adopt a healthier eating plan as soon as possible. It will significantly improve not only your appearance but also your state of health.

PUT YOUR GOALS IN PERSPECTIVE

Are our efforts to lose weight at any cost really worthwhile? Paintings by Rubens, Raphael, and Renoir allow us to appreciate the sight of a beautiful and voluptuous woman. During the era when these painters lived, a thin woman symbolized poverty, inferior status, and disease, and therefore was not suitable to serve as a painter's model. Even Lord Byron, who himself was one of the first poets to go on a crash diet, thought that thin women were not beautiful and compared them to withered butterflies.

In modern times, the tables have turned and thinness has become the symbol of beauty and of being "in." This is evident in a comparative survey that examined the weight of the winners of the Miss America Pageant. At first, the BMIs of the participants in the Miss America Pageant were between 20 and 25—optimal by today's standards. Over the years, it has dropped to less than 18.5—that's underweight even by today's standards.

The BMI of the "fattest" Miss America (Rosemary LaPlanche of California), in the year 1941, was 22.4, whereas that of the thinnest (Susan Akin of Mississippi), in 1986, was 16.9—a candidate for hospitalization, according to this index. Since no dramatic increase in height occurred during those years, we can attribute the decreased BMI to a drop in weight.

THE BREAD FOR LIFE DIET allows for gradual weight loss, a gradual drop in the percentage of body fat, and a significant drop in waist circumference, leading to overall health improvement.

3

It's All in Your Head

The brain is more than just another organ of the body. It comprises our essence, personality, and reactions as well as our mental and emotional capacity. Everything we do, feel, think, and fantasize about comes from the brain.

The brain contains billions of cells called neurons, which transmit information nonstop 24/7 at lightning speed. Like busy librarians, the neurons constantly retrieve information from all over the body, which the brain interprets as feelings and sensations like anger, pain, sexual desire, heat, cold, and, of course, hunger and satiety. The brain then uses electrical signals and chemical substances to distribute these sensations throughout the body.

In some ways, the brain is similar to a wizard in his workshop, producing specific "potions" for specific effects. Though scientists have identified only a very small number of these substances, we know there are love "potions," (phenylethylamine), excitement "potions" (dopamine), calming "potions" (serotonin), pain-relieving "potions"(endorphins), and hunger and satiety "potions" (serotonin and neuropeptide Y), among others. *The Bread for Life Diet* is based on, among other things, the role of serotonin as a satiety and calming potion.

HOW YOUR BRAIN MAKES YOU FAT

The potions that trigger sensations of satiety (the feeling of fullness we get after eating) and of hunger are secreted mainly by the part of the brain known as the hypothalamus. The size of a small plum, the hypothalamus not only regulates hunger-satiety, but also body temperature, the emotions of anger and fear, body fluid balance, and mating and sexual behavior, just to name a few. In a nutshell, it is responsible for various issues associated with survival. That's why, during prehistoric times, the hypothalamus was one of the first parts of the brain to develop in animals.

The cell clusters that make up the hunger/satiety centers in the hypothalamus get their signals from different parts of the body, mainly adipose (fat) tissues, the pancreas, the liver, the stomach, and the gut. Depending on the signal, these cell clusters respond by producing substances that either turn on hunger or turn on satiety. So, contrary to what many people think, the origin of hunger and satiety is not in the stomach but in the brain.

The existence of these cell clusters was discovered in the 1960s through experiments with animals such as rats and roosters, which involved deliberate injury to targeted areas of their brains. The scientists found that trauma to a particular part of the hypothalamus caused the animals to refuse food, even to the point of dying from starvation. They defined this area of the brain as the "hunger center." Injuries to another part of the hypothalamus caused animals to eat constantly, which led to pathological and sometimes fatal weight gain. This area was dubbed the "satiety center."

Since then, researchers have made the same observations in people who were injured in accidents. As a result, we now know that the brain contains hunger and satiety centers that are made up of various types of cells and secrete substances, called neuropeptides, that affect, among other activities, human eating behavior. So far, scientists have discovered more than a dozen neuropeptides and others, no doubt, will be discovered. A thriving diet industry, which drives the development of drugs for controlling obesity, is constantly looking for formulas that can be used to affect neuropeptides and cause deliberate weight loss or weight gain.

BALANCE IS EVERYTHING

The physiological role of the hunger-satiety mechanism is to maintain a normal fixed weight. It is essential to every living creature's ability to survive. The hunger center, in response to the absence of food, produces potions that can urge an animal (or a human) to travel long distances in search of food, without concern for danger or fatigue. Eating causes the stomach to expand, liver and fat tissues to fill with nutrients, and blood sugar levels to rise, all triggering the brain to secrete potions that give the signal to stop eating. This mechanism is important for preventing obesity.

In nature, an obese animal has a lower chance of survival because extra weight will slow it down and reduce its ability to gather food. It also becomes easy prey for predators. The same mechanism is also important for preventing weight loss, as an animal that is too thin would quickly become tired and weak, also making it unlikely to survive.

In wild animals, the activity of the hunger and satiety centers is balanced:

They eat when they are hungry and stop eating when they are full. A tiger that kills a deer eats only until it is full and leaves the remains for other animals. Unfortunately, the same harmony between hunger and satiety is rarely evidenced in 21st century humans. We know that it exists because we can see it in babies. Even if a mother and grandmother stand on their heads and plead, a baby who is full will not continue eating. Likewise, a hungry baby won't stop crying until fed. Puppies that haven't been spoiled by their loving owners eat until they are full and then dig a hole in which they hide their remaining food.

The harmony between hunger and satiety in adult human beings, however, has become disrupted by our society of abundance. The 21st century sees only a relatively small number of people eating primarily from hunger. The majority have other reasons for eating, including anger, boredom, fatigue, and frustration as well as holidays, celebrations, and social gatherings.

SIMPLE IS BEST

One way to restore the balance between hunger and satiety is by eating "simple" but tasty foods—the hallmark of *The Bread for Life Diet*. By that, I mean food that is cooked without being drenched in spices or sauces. Why? When a meal is simple and less varied, we eat less. That's what scientists found when they performed several interesting laboratory experiments with rats, which, like most wild animals, have a normal hunger-satiety balance.

In the experiments, one set of rats was fed popular snacks, such as smoked meats, hard cheeses, and potato chips. Researchers called this the "Cafeteria Diet." Another set of rats was fed ordinary monotonous rat chow. The rats fed the Cafeteria Diet ate more than the rats given ordinary rat chow, and it was no surprise that they gained weight. The experiments clearly demonstrated how the abundance and availability of food in the Western diet lead to overindulgence. The results indicate that even for animals that normally maintain a good hunger-satiety balance, eating rich, spicy, and, most important, varied foods of the Western diet disrupts the balance in the hunger-satiety centers of the animals' brains, often leading to increased food intake and weight gain. By contrast, less-rich and less-varied food balances consumption and permits better control of the amounts eaten.

The same process takes place in humans. Take steak, for example. How much steak can an average person eat if it isn't dripping in sauce and isn't flanked by potatoes and buttered mushrooms? What about pasta? How many noodles can an average person eat if they're served simply with a fresh tomato sauce? On the other hand, if meat is added to the sauce and the pasta is covered with Parmesan cheese, one is more likely to gorge oneself (remember the Cafeteria Diet?).

The challenge is that simple food can be hard to come by, especially in restaurants and at social gatherings. Meals serve both as a form of enter-tainment and status in our lives, whether at home or dining out. People who host dinner parties in their homes often like to impress their guests with their wonderful culinary skills, so they wouldn't dream of making a plain, simple dish. Many people come from families in which holidays are centered on food—vast quantities of food. Traditionally, it is the way the family hostess, often the mother, grandmother, sister, or mother-in-law, expresses her love for her family. The rest of the family responds in kind by eating and eating without leaving a crumb behind. Even if they feel about to burst, everyone suddenly has room for dessert when it arrives, as if someone waved a magic wand. No one wants to insult the hostess! It's no wonder that just after the holidays, the magazines are filled with diet tips and doctors' offices are filled with sick people.

In many ways, eating in a restaurant presents similar challenges. Those who prefer to eat out will rarely select a simple dish that they could pre-pare in their own kitchens. It's not why they get dressed up, hire a babysitter, and bring along lots of money!

In the end, however, what you eat is not up to the hostess at your holiday party or the chef in the restaurant. It's up to you. And the rule to go by is "simple is always best." By "simple" I do not mean tasteless and unappealing. There is no ban on cooking delicacies on *The Bread for Life Diet*, so long as you don't smother them with sauces or butter. And you can still enjoy a full meal, even if it doesn't consist of multiple courses.

A FEAST FOR THE SENSES

Naturally, you want to eat food that smells good, looks good, and tastes good! You want to eat food you love. Food appeal is a personal thing because it begins in an individual's senses, which are driven by smell, sight, and taste. Stimulating these senses intensifies the desire to eat. If you use your senses properly, you can use them to your advantage and eat less.

Taste

The sense of taste is initiated in the taste buds, located on the surface of the tongue. It responds to only a specific number of flavors—sweet, salty, sour, bitter, and a recently discovered taste called *umami*, which is produced from a substance called glutamate, found in meat. Its familiar derivative, monosodium glutamate, is what gives Chinese cuisine its unique flavor.

Taste buds are made up of cells that are distributed across the surface of the tongue, with concentrations located on specific parts of the tongue. Cells that are receptive to a salty taste are concentrated mostly on the tip and sides of the tongue; cells that are receptive to bitter are at the base of the tongue; cells that are receptive to sweet are at the front and toward the middle of the tongue; and cells that are receptive to sour are on the sides of the tongue.

In order for the tongue to extract flavors fully, food must be wet and chewed. The phrase "melts in your mouth" says it all. Ice cream is most delicious when it melts in your mouth, not when it's still frozen. Meat chewed and swallowed hurriedly is virtually tasteless. Chewing slowly and completely gets the full flavor out of food, which contributes to the feeling of satiety. So the more you chew, the fuller you feel.

Taste perception varies from one person to another, as does the number of taste cells each person has. That's why some people enjoy Roquefort cheese and some find it repulsive. Other factors influence taste as well. For example, taste dulls with age, which is one reason people often eat less as they reach their senior years.

Smell

If there are only five flavors, where does our extreme enjoyment of food come from? How do the variety of flavors become so rich—from the wonders of French cuisine to the delicacies of the Far East? The answer is the sense of smell, which enhances the various nuances inherent in each flavor. People who have no sense of smell do not enjoy their food. In fact, anyone who has ever had a stuffy nose knows how flavorless and unappetizing food can be and how quickly flavor and enjoyment return when the sense of smell returns.

Sight

The sense of sight also plays a major role in the taste process. The eyes are often the first to send signals to the brain that the taste buds are in for a treat. How many times have you found yourself peering into the refrigerator in the middle of the night because you saw an enticing meal on a commercial? This is another example that senses—not necessarily hunger—prompt us to eat.

The senses are intensely tied to our ability to make food choices. This is important to know because you can use your senses to avoid situations that lead good intentions astray.

Your sense of taste lures you to buy a *second* hot dog from your favorite hot dog stand. Your sense of smell lowers your resistance for a certain dessert as soon as you step through the door of your favorite restaurant or pass by the neighborhood bakery. Your sense of sight is powerful enough to cause you to salivate as you peruse the full-color photographs in a food magazine.

THE ROLE OF CONDITIONING

It's not only our senses that pique our appetite. Our thoughts, imagination, and associations also play a role. Pavlov's famous experiments with dogs demonstrate how this works. In these experiments, the secretion of saliva and gastric juices was noted, first in response to feeding accompanied by the sound of a bell, and afterward, in response to the sound of the bell alone. It came as a surprise to Pavlov that digestive juices were secreted in response to the seemingly neutral stimulus of the bell ringing, even when no food was given. Pavlov called this phenomenon "conditioned reflex."

Our behavior in general and our eating behavior in particular are based on many such conditioned reflexes and habits. Take, for example, the common habit of eating something tasty, like a doughnut, with coffee or tea. "It's just not the same without it," is a statement many of us can identify with. But what constitutes "something tasty?" Generally it's a doughnut, cookies, a slice of cake, or the like—something sweet. In other words, people who are conditioned into this habit believe that they can't really enjoy drinking coffee without eating a sweet baked good along with it. Little things like this can add up to a lot of weight gain over time.

One of the important goals of every diet is to neutralize conditioned behavior—in our example, to separate the coffee from the doughnuts, so to speak. If a woman has a fight with her husband, for example, she may immediately turn to a container of ice cream for comfort. Pounds are added with every fight because the ice cream becomes an inseparable part of the ritual. The moment the wife understands that a fight with her husband is only a fight with her husband, and that ice cream has no role in resolving it, fighting will no longer be a trigger for gaining weight. If she is aware that it is just a conditioned reflex, she can consciously switch to an alternative conditioning—something pleasant—like taking a walk or going shopping. She can even share the understanding and the new ritual with her husband, so that they can walk together and use that time to reconcile their differences. You can use the same technique to learn to identify the situations that trigger your raids on the refrigerator.

A common conditioned behavior among men is watching sports on television, whether alone or with company, outfitted with beer and a full supply of snacks. During the game, no mouth is ever idle—and not just because they are yelling at the game on TV!

Our conditioned behaviors coupled with the ever-present influence of our senses can lead us to overeat much of the time. That's not to say that our senses serve a bad purpose. Quite the opposite. Our senses were really developed to encourage our enjoyment of food. It is only when we don't pay attention to them in the way they were intended that we run into trouble.

Pavlov, again, can be used to explain this. He found that the brain can use the senses of sight and smell to initiate the cephalic (meaning "head" in Greek) phase of the digestive process even before food touches the tongue. Like Pavlov's dogs, human beings go through a cephalic phase. The cephalic phase is important because it is necessary to the sense of satiety. Most people don't experience satiety because of bad eating habits. We eat while watching TV, working at our desks, or reading a book. We eat while concentrating on something else rather than on the food itself. As a result, we do not reach the same level of satiety or we reach it only after we have consumed far too much food. If you concentrate on what you are eating, you can eat less and enjoy the food more.

RECONDITION YOUR EATING HABITS

Bad eating habits, most of which are only conditioned reflexes, are most often what differentiates a person who wants to lose weight from a person who successfully loses weight. We must break the conditioned response and get in tune with the cephalic phase of eating. If you concentrate on the experience of enjoying your meal, it will help you break the old habits that may be causing you to put on weight, and then get in tune with the cephalic phase of eating. Here is what you should do:

Concentrate on the food you are eating.

If you observe the eating habits of pets or animals in the zoo, you will notice that they are so absorbed in their food that they ignore everything else that is going on around them. They do not want to be disturbed. And when they are, watch out! Even a pet dog can turn on you if you disturb it while it is eating.

Humans are just the opposite. We eat in front of the television or the computer, while reading a book, and while holding an engaging conversation at the table. In doing so, we do not derive full benefit from the cephalic phase—the stage when we should be concentrating on the food we are eating. As a result, we do not benefit from the part of the process that significantly contributes to a sense of satiety. This makes us prone to eat more than we really need to and to do so without giving it a second thought, and without fully enjoying it! So, when you eat, *concentrate only on the food*. Eat at a table and not in places that are not meant for eating, such as in front of the television, at your desk, or while driving to work or to a meeting. Disorganized eating prevents us from concentrating on our food and using the cephalic phase to our full advantage.

Respect both your food and yourself.

When we eat in a respectful and organized manner, preferably in a pleasant atmosphere, we eat less and feel fuller. Let's compare what happens at two different kinds of restaurants, one family-style and one French gourmet. At a family restaurant with a dinner buffet and salad bar, we pile huge portions on our plates, try two or three different kinds of bread smothered with butter, go back for second and third servings, and top the meal off with dessert. At a French restaurant, on the other hand, we are served small portions on elegant dishes and time is allowed between each course for us to converse without interrupting our eating. This kind of dining also encourages us to eat more slowly, with respect and concentration. We then use the cephalic phase to maximum effect and consequently feel completely satiated, tranquil, and satisfied by a smaller meal.

Make the experience a pleasure.

Sit at the table, select beautiful silverware, serve the food on attractive dinnerware, eat slowly, and enjoy every bite. When we eat in style, respect the food, and make it attractive, we eat less. It is a conditioned response well worth adopting.

Chew your food slowly and completely.

Feel the food texture and really taste the flavor. By chewing your food thoroughly, you will enjoy the taste more, eat less, and feel fuller. A person who eats quickly does not take full advantage of the cephalic phase. Moreover, when eating with others, he or she finishes his meal before everyone else and has to take a second or even a third helping in order to avoid sitting around waiting for the others to finish.

Consider your portion size before starting to eat it.

Most people finish whatever portion is served to them. Given the choice to enlarge the portion size, especially at a discount, most people opt to take the larger portion. And they eat all they paid for regardless of whether less food would have been enough to make them feel full and satisfied. This so-called "super-sizing" phenomenon is currently considered a significant reasons for overweight and obesity.

We are accustomed to finishing what is on the plate. The larger the portion size, the more we eat, usually without even paying any attention. To demonstrate this, volunteers were given a portion of pasta once a week for 4 weeks. Each time, they were given a larger portion. When given increased portions, the volunteers simply ate more, and only a few of them even noticed that the portions were changing. All reported that they were satisfied each time they finished their meal, no matter what the portion size.

In another experiment, college students were given soup. Some of the portions were served in regular bowls, whereas others were served in special bowls fitted with a tube that gradually refilled the bowls as the students ate. The students with the special bowls kept on eating. The results of these and similar experiments show that the larger the portion, the more we eat.

Here's what you can do to fight this impulse:

◆ When you are served a portion, choose *in advance* how much of it you are going to eat, and leave the rest on your plate, no matter what anyone says. It's *your* health and shape.

◆ When you choose your portion size, opt for the smallest one that you think will satisfy your hunger. If, after finishing it, you're still hungry, drink a glass or two of nonsugared nonalcoholic beverage, and wait approximately 20 minutes. If you're still hungry, get a second helping. Even if it costs you a little more, it's well worth the attempt to avoid overeating.

Do your grocery shopping when you're full.

The cephalic phase has an effect even when you are buying food. When you go grocery shopping on an empty stomach, you buy foods you don't need or want, like fattening treats. I am sure you've heard this before. Everyone knows not to food shop on an empty stomach but they do it anyway. This is not a good idea! Grabbing something to eat on your way out the door won't work either. Plan your food shopping for after lunch or dinner. Guaranteed, you won't buy as much—and you'll save some money, too.

THE BREAD FOR LIFE DIET is based on the brain's role in controlling the hunger-satiety centers in your brain. It provides you with practical tools for controlling hunger through food choices and portion sizes.

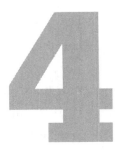

Serotonin & Weight Loss

One of the most important discoveries in obesity research was the basic understanding of the important role serotonin plays in the human hunger and satiety cycle. Serotonin, a neurotransmitter secreted by the hypothalamus, affects our daily lives in many ways: It is involved in mood, appetite, sleep, blood pressure, response to pain, sexuality, and even in how we perceive the outside world. Research is only beginning to understand the various effects serotonin has on the mind and body, but it is well-established that it has a strong effect on hunger and satiety. Thus its important tie to *The Bread for Life Diet*.

Serotonin research began during the 1970s when scientists observed an increase in suicides and in people requiring psychiatric help due to depression in Northern European countries, where there was little daytime light during winter. The scientists found a correlation among these human behaviors and levels of serotonin, which sharply drops during the long, dark days of winter. These kinds of psychiatric disorders became known as Seasonal Affective Disorders (SAD). One treatment technique that was developed was to increase serotonin production through the use of full-spectrum lights that could mimic natural light. But the scientists also made another observation among people with SAD: They had a tendency to put on weight during winter, which was the trigger that sent researchers searching for a link between serotonin and obesity. Since then, a lot of research on animals and humans has been performed revealing how food affects the brain production of serotonin and how serotonin affects food choices.

One noteworthy discovery was the ability of carbohydrates to raise the levels of serotonin in the brain. Later on, researchers discovered something even more interesting—that eating a protein meal sharply decreases the serotonin level. I was involved in this research and was initially quite surprised by it. This finding helps explain in part why high-protein diets are so difficult to sustain. A low serotonin level causes craving for sweets and, eventually, people break their diets. This led me to the understanding that we can influence serotonin levels through varying the ratio of carbohydrates and proteins.

THE UPS AND DOWNS OF SEROTONIN

Serotonin level tests in humans are not performed routinely and are used mainly for research purposes. One reason is that specialists still debate whether the costly blood test is precise enough to accurately reflect serotonin levels in the brain. Normal blood levels of serotonin fall within a broad range, and even when it is very low, this doesn't indicate a *disease.* Only a very excessive level can be indicative of a disease state or health complication.

Many factors can affect your serotonin level, for example:

✦ Eating carbohydrates—raises serotonin level.

✦ Eating proteins—decreases serotonin level.

✦ Gender—on average, women have a lower serotonin level than men.

✦ Seasonal changes—serotonin level decreases during the winter, when sunlight is weaker and days are shorter.

✦ Sex hormones—serotonin level decreases in the middle of the menstrual cycle during ovulation, a few days before each period, and during menopause.

A low serotonin level can cause bad moods, depression, a low threshold for pain, headaches, memory lapses, concentration problems, restless sleep, insomnia, daytime drowsiness, and—here is an important dieting factor—a craving for carbohydrates, especially sweets.

HOW CARBS TURN OFF HUNGER

Eating carbohydrates actually raises serotonin levels. Here's why: Serotonin is made up of an amino acid called tryptophan. To produce serotonin, tryptophan must pass through a "frontier" in the brain, called the Blood-Brain Barrier, or BBB, consisting of delicate passages between the ends of the blood vessels and the brain's internal membranes. This barrier, which isolates the brain from the body, ensures that undesirable and harmful substances don't pass into this most vital and protected of the body's organs. It allows in only substances the brain requires for proper functioning. It is not always easy for tryptophan to get through the BBB because it competes with other amino acids that can push tryptophan aside to gain entry. Only

THE SOCIAL SIDE OF SEROTONIN

In addition to the physiological factors that affect serotonin levels, there are indications that social factors also have an impact, though studies have been carried out only on animals.

In one experiment, two deer were incited to fight each other. Serotonin levels dropped in the animal that lost and increased in the animal that won. In another study, serotonin levels were examined among a species of monkeys that live in family groups. The monkeys with lower social status had low serotonin levels, whereas the serotonin levels of the leaders of the "family" were high.

Lower average serotonin levels among women compared to men is usually explained by their hormonal differences. But one unproven hypothesis among sociologists, based on these animal studies, suggests that this phenomenon is actually the result of the lower social status of women experienced throughout the ages. This makes me believe that in an era in which women achieve and attain a high social status, their average serotonin levels will rise. What a wonderful incentive to work toward that goal!

when competing amino acids are successfully diverted away from the BBB is tryptophan able to enter the brain and participate in serotonin production.

This diversion is performed with the help of the hormone insulin, which detours competing amino acids into the muscles. Rising levels of insulin give tryptophan, which is far less affected by insulin, an open gateway into the brain. Since tryptophan's entry into the brain depends on a rise in insulin level, foods that make insulin levels go up will obviously raise serotonin levels as well. What foods are these? Those containing carbohydrates!

Because serotonin is made up of an amino acid, it would seem logical to assume that eating proteins (consisting of amino acids) would promote the production of serotonin. However, this is not what happens. When we eat proteins, the gateway to the brain becomes flooded with competing amino acids. As a result, tryptophan doesn't stand a chance of gaining entry into the brain. Because tryptophan is needed to manufacture serotonin, the level of serotonin in the brain drops. This explains why so many people who follow a protein-based diet often feel the symptoms of low serotonin levels, including irritability, insomnia, poor concentration, and depression. I have had many women patients come to me after being on protein diets who say how nervous they had been, how they had yelled at their children and husbands, and how relationships had been damaged.

SWEETS AND HUNGER

The decrease in serotonin also explains the strong desire for something sweet after consuming a generous portion of steak (protein).

Eating carbohydrates raises serotonin. The fastest-acting ones are *simple* carbohydrates, such as sugars, chocolate, candy, crackers, and foods containing refined flour. Most packaged foods are loaded with them. When you eat them, your serotonin level rises quickly. Sounds good, right? Unfortunately, there's a catch: Following the rapid rise in serotonin comes an equally rapid drop. Within an hour or less, we once again feel an intense need for sweets. This is how the sweet cycle begins, and over time, it becomes increasingly difficult to break. Considering that most sweets are rich in calories, this cycle causes weight gain. By contrast, when you eat slower-acting *complex* carbohydrates, such as bread or pasta, the rise in your serotonin level is more moderate, but it lasts longer—approximately 3 to 4 hours.

This, in a nutshell, explains the basis of my diet and the importance of eating small carbohydrate meals every 3 to 4 hours. It helps keep your serotonin level relatively constant and prevents it from crashing.

HIGH-PROTEIN DIETS: WOMEN UNFRIENDLY

Here is a question for women on a high-protein diet: Do you feel nervous, exhausted, or ready to start crying for no apparent reason? Are you shouting at people, sleeping badly, craving for anything sweet or for a piece of bread? It turns out that there is a good reason for it: Not only is the average serotonin level in women relatively low (compared to men) but eating proteins lowers it still further. That's why high-protein diets are not women friendly. Most women need carbohydrates to feel good and function well.

THE SEROTONIN-HUNGER CONNECTION

All of this suggests that craving carbohydrates is the brain's physiological way to get a rise in serotonin level. Without doubt, there are also psychological and behavioral reasons why we crave sweets, such as the need to pamper and comfort ourselves and our need for immediate gratification, which are also very important (as explained in Chapter 2). I believe, though, that understanding the basic physiological process in the brain is as important as understanding the psychological nature of overeating. It is also a key to freeing ourselves from the feelings of guilt that usually accompany our overindulgence in sweets. Knowing all this helps us make smart choices in the way we eat.

When we don't eat for many hours, the serotonin level drops, which triggers the production of hunger potions by the hypothalamus. The sudden flood of hunger potions in the brain makes us feel overcome with hunger. Given the option of relieving this feeling by choosing from a variety of foods, most of us choose sweet snacks. Now we understand why: because sweets are fast at raising the serotonin level. Moreover, it is the easiest option—just tear open the package, and that's it. No preparation, no cooking, not even a dish gets dirty.

When we eat sweets, we increase the serotonin level for a short time, after which it goes down and we crave more and more. When we eat proteins, the serotonin level decreases very quickly, and we crave sweets again. Welcome to the "sweet cycle!" When we are in this cycle, we can become absolutely frenzied in our eating: munching sweets, then salty things, and then sweets again. After indulging, we find ourselves feeling guilty, sad, and regretful, and to console ourselves, we completely pig out.

That being the case, how can we get out of the sweet cycle? How can we raise and maintain our serotonin level in order to control our eating habits?

Antidepressants such as Prozac™ and its newer generations are based on improving the brain's serotonin activity. Although *The Bread for Life Diet* doesn't claim to be a cure for clinical depression, it can certainly complement the drug therapy given to people suffering from this disease. By contrast, a high-protein diet is liable to increase the severity of the disease.

MAINTAINING HIGH SEROTONIN

As explained earlier, eating *simple* carbohydrates (sugars) quickly raises serotonin levels, but these levels drop just as quickly. Eating *complex* carbohydrates also raises serotonin levels, but more moderately, and keeps the level high for 3 to 4 hours. When serotonin is at a higher level, you don't feel hungry, and that is one of the keys to *The Bread for Life Diet.* When you eat *complex* carbohydrates every 3 to 4 hours, you don't feel hungry and you don't have cravings. The hunger and misery typical of weight-loss diets do not exist.

By eating complex carbohydrates every 3 to 4 hours, you achieve several goals:

- ✦ Serotonin level rises.

- ✦ Serotonin level remains at a higher level for longer periods and is not given the opportunity to drop before your next meal, thereby preventing hunger and especially a craving for sweet foods.

- ✦ You enjoy an ongoing feeling of satiety and calm.

- ✦ Dividing your daily food into many small meals, so that you always have something to eat, gives you the feeling of security—there is no fear that you will starve for the rest of the day.

- ✦ Your body does not go into starvation mode, meaning your metabolism does not slow down in order to economize and you therefore can continue to lose weight.

- ✦ You don't feel hungry, so you don't feel like attacking your next meal as if you are starving. This means you can eat more slowly. As a result, you eat far fewer calories, enjoy your food more, and consequently lose weight.

- ✦ You don't crave bread and other complex carbohydrates because you already have them at almost every meal.

Does that sound like dieting? I have had thousands of patients who say "not at all!"

While it is true that you will need to sacrifice that chocolate bar and other sweets you love so dearly, it will be much less of a problem than you imagine. Many of the chocolate lovers on *The Bread for Life Diet* tell me how surprised they are that they don't have a single craving for chocolate for weeks. They never dreamed it could happen.

One woman said at our first meeting: "I can give up all the food; I am absolutely sure I can't give up chocolate." After a week on *The Bread for Life Diet*, she said: "I am shocked: I still don't believe I haven't had even a single chocolate bar this week. I just didn't need any." At the last meeting, she said: "I can look at the cakes in the coffee shop and remain uninterested, even when my husband prompts me to have one. I can take just a bite from his dessert and stop at that."

THIN MEN ARE DIFFERENT

Not everyone is attracted to sweet foods. There are those who would actually prefer a juicy steak. Most of these people have high serotonin levels. Food preference tests have revealed that most thin men prefer to eat proteins such as meat and fish while most women, both overweight and thin, and overweight men, prefer carbohydrates.

A young girl who loved cake said after starting *The Bread for Life Diet*: "I didn't believe I could live without having a piece of cake a few times a day. Now I can manage with one piece a week and feel fine."

The most amazing thing is that as long as my patients keep eating every 3 to 4 hours, they lose and maintain their weight. The moment they stop it and go back to eating three or fewer meals a day, they regain weight. Serotonin is a strong potion!

People with a low serotonin level usually look tired, feel drained, and are slow in their responses. One of the female patients who came to me wanting to lose weight was so slow, tired, and unfocused at our first meeting that she stopped talking in mid-sentence because she had forgotten what she had started to say. When I asked her what she ate, she was quick to answer: "Only sweet things. I really don't need food. I eat only sweet things. It keeps me alert and makes me feel good." After just 2 weeks on *The Bread for Life Diet*, her mood improved, her eyes sparkled, her fatigue disappeared, and her alertness was restored. By the end of the treatment, she had lost nearly 55 pounds, felt terrific, and had renewed energy to take life by storm.

As I've already said, a low serotonin level is not a disease, and there is no medical treatment for it. It might better be likened to low blood pressure: it's unpleasant, it's tiring, there is no medicine to take for it, and you have to learn to live with it. In the case of a low serotonin level, feeling better is possible with the help of *The Bread for Life Diet*.

THE BREAD FOR LIFE DIET is based on the effect of serotonin on the hunger and satiety processes in the brain. When serotonin is high, as happens when you eat a bread-based or *complex* carbohydrate meal, you feel calm and full. Elevated serotonin levels will prevent you from craving sweets.

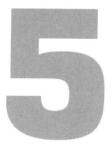

5

Insulin & Weight Gain

Insulin, a hormone made and secreted by the pancreas, plays a decisive role in weight gain. Here is what happens: When we eat, the level of sugar in the blood rises. That triggers the pancreas to release insulin, which is responsible for moving nutrients—mainly a sugar called glucose—from the bloodstream into body cells, mainly in muscle and fat tissues, where they are used as fuel and as building materials to keep cells functioning normally. As insulin causes sugar to get into the cells, the blood glucose level drops, and the insulin level returns to normal. In other words, insulin decreases blood glucose level. Among healthy people, this cycle—from eating the meal to getting the insulin level back to normal—takes about 2 to 3 hours.

TOO MUCH OF A GOOD THING

In many people, especially those who are overweight, insulin levels are often higher than normal, even after not eating for many hours, and rise further after a meal. That means that insulin levels do not return to normal, even for many hours after a meal. These people walk around with abnormally high levels of insulin for most of the day, usually without even being aware of it. This condition is known as hyperinsulinemia and has a great impact on the development of obesity and of type 2 diabetes.

During the early stages of hyperinsulinemia, people often experience what we call hypoglycemia—a sudden decrease in the level of glucose in the blood. This is understandable, because the role of insulin is to lower the blood glucose level. At this stage, hyperinsulinemia can cause dizziness, trembling, sweating, and even fainting. However, over time, the body's tissues get used to the excess insulin and develop resistance to it. According to statistics, about 40 percent of the apparently healthy adult population has different degrees of hyperinsulinemia and insulin resistance. These numbers are even higher among the overweight and the obese.

In one of my research groups, consisting of people weighing an average of 273 pounds, 60 percent had insulin levels above normal. After 4 months on *The Bread for Life Diet*, their insulin levels decreased significantly. In many of them, insulin levels even went back to normal.

Here, in a nutshell, is how this process works: Insulin acts as a key that opens the door to body cells so they can take in sugar. If cells are overexposed to insulin for prolonged periods, however, they become less sensitive to its effects and more and more insulin is necessary to gain entry. This means that the pancreas, which manufactures insulin, has to work harder. As a result, it eventually gets "worn down" to the point where it is unable to produce enough insulin to get the job done. This means blood glucose levels rise and, in the course of time, can become dangerously high. In other words, diabetes develops.

This explains the strong and significant link between obesity, hyperinsulinemia, and diabetes. Scientists have even coined a new word for it: *diabesity*. It also explains why type 2 diabetes, which usually develops in adulthood (often called adult-onset diabetes), is now being diagnosed more and more in children. The cause is the frightening increase in childhood obesity.

Hyperinsulinemia impacts weight for several reasons:

✦ Genetically, fat accumulation is our most important survival mechanism. Insulin is an anabolic, or body-building, hormone, so a person with hyperinsulinemia (that is, too much insulin) finds it difficult to lose weight because insulin prevents fat tissues from breaking down. It is a survival mechanism.

✦ Hyperinsulinemia increases appetite in general and stimulates an intense demand for sweet foods in particular, especially after a full, hearty meal. People commonly describe the feeling as having "a hole in the stomach that must be filled."

✦ Insulin resistance and hyperinsulinemia interfere with the normal production of serotonin, a key brain chemical that plays a key role in appetite suppression.

✦ People with hyperinsulinemia burn off fewer calories during physical activity than do people without hyperinsulinemia.

Hyperinsulinemia also contributes to the risk of developing what is known as metabolic syndrome (also called syndrome X), a compendium of disorders that include high blood pressure, diabetes, and elevated triglycerides and cholesterol in the blood, all risk factors that can lead to heart disease and stroke. Metabolic syndrome involves a fatty liver, gout, and sub-clinical inflammation. It is characterized by abdominal, apple-shape obesity. In this type of obesity, fat tissue is accumulated both inside the abdominal area (visceral fat—"viscera" is Latin for major internal organ) and under the skin (subcutaneous fat). There is clear evidence that visceral fat poses a greater health risk than subcutaneous fat in both men and women, even if they are not otherwise overweight. That's because abdominal fat produces different kinds of active substances, such as cytokines, which cause sub-clinical inflammation, blood-clotting abnormalities, and other blood-flow-related problems that are believed to be risk factors for cardiovascular disease.

As explained in Chapter 2, it is easy to determine if you have this type of obesity. Simply measure your waist. If it exceeds 41 inches for a man or 35 inches for a woman, you fit the description. Losing weight and decreasing waist size is the best way to address high insulin levels, improve insulin sensitivity, and decrease the risks of metabolic syndrome.

A state of hyperinsulinemia can exist undetected (and thus untreated) for years. In most cases, it will lead to diabetes—hence its other name: pre-diabetes. As I've mentioned, it is much more difficult for people with hyperinsulinemia to lose weight and all too easy for them to gain weight than it is for people (even obese people) who do not have the condition. Sadly, people who are unaware that they have hyperinsulinemia—as is the case with most of them—are subject to suffering beyond the sheer burden of their obesity. They are often ridiculed for lacking willpower and character, when in fact that may not be the case. They describe their attempts at weight loss as feeling as if they are running into a brick wall. Having encountered many such people in my clinic, I understand their frustration and can help relieve their suffering by explaining their problem and putting them on *The Bread for Life Diet*, which helps tremendously.

Though some hormones, like catecholamines, stress hormones, and steroids, also factor into the development of obesity and interfere with losing weight, they are not affected as strongly as insulin is by the food we eat. A few doctors have started prescribing anti-diabetic drugs to people with hyperinsulinemia. This improves insulin levels and, together with diet and physical activity, can help in postponing the development of diabetes.

There is no magic cure for overweight and obesity and no medicine without side effects. *The Bread for Life Diet* may be as close as real life gets in terms of an easy and effective solution. This diet, coupled with physical exercise, lowers insulin and sugar levels, increases sensitivity to insulin, facilitates weight loss, and prevents the development of diseases associated with metabolic syndrome.

INSULIN AND THE BREAD FOR LIFE DIET

Both overweight and obesity can lead to or be caused by hyperinsulinemia, which makes for a vicious cycle: hyperinsulinemia—overweight—more hyperinsulinemia—more overweight.

The Bread for Life Diet helps you break this cycle.

When trying to lose weight, you need to keep your insulin levels as close to normal as possible at all times. There are two major things that work against this goal: Eating sweet foods (simple carbohydrates) and eating big, heavy meals.

Conversely, there are two major things that work toward this goal: Avoiding sweet foods and eating small meals, distributed over the entire day.

That's where The Bread for Life Diet comes in: Eating small meals of *complex* carbohydrates spread evenly throughout the day automatically helps you avoid sweets and heavy meals and perfectly addresses both the insulin and serotonin issues.

THE GLYCEMIC INDEX

Eating any kind of food, but carbohydrates in particular, raises the level of glucose, and consequently insulin, in the blood. But how high those levels go depends on the composition of the individual food. Foods that significantly raise glucose levels will make it more difficult to lose weight, and those that cause a smaller rise in glucose will make it easier to lose weight.

A measure called "glycemic index" indicates the relative rise in blood glucose level in response to consuming various foods that contain carbohydrates. It is measured against the rise that occurs after consuming white bread, or glucose. The index was computed on the basis of the average blood glucose response of many people to a variety of different foods and designates an average value for each food. Foods that greatly increase glucose and insulin levels get a higher index value. These are the foods that make it more difficult to lose weight, whereas foods with a low glycemic index value make it easier. Naturally, if you want to lose weight, you should generally choose foods with a low glycemic index for your everyday consumption.

Research on the effect of carbohydrates on raising blood glucose resulted in yet another measure called glycemic *load*. This measure takes into consideration the serving size as well as the amount of carbohydrates (excluding dietary fiber) in a food. Using it, however, is somewhat more complex, so I prefer the relative simplicity of the glycemic index, especially since research has not yet determined which measure is more significant.

The glycemic indexes of various foods are generally measured against either white bread set at a value of 100 or against glucose set at value of 100. White-bread-based and glucose-based glycemic index values are different (white-bread-based values are about 40 percent higher). This book uses white-bread-based values.

INSULIN: WHO'S IN THE RESISTANCE?

Hyperinsulinemia is probably one of the most underdiagnosed metabolic conditions contributing to weight gain today. It is a shame, too, because diagnosis is the first step toward successfully winning at weight loss and preventing diabetes.

During my work as a clinical dietitian, I have seen thousands of obese and overweight people with hyperinsulinemia, many of whom were able to reverse their condition and achieve successful weight loss. I have treated so many people with the problem that I can predict the likelihood that they have it just by seeing them and talking to them. Excess fat around the middle, family history, history of struggling to lose weight, signs of hypoglycemia, craving for sweets after big meals, and tiredness are among the symptoms. But it is never a sure diagnosis until it is confirmed by a blood test.

If you suspect this could be your problem, you should ask your doctor to order the relevant tests. There are a few different ways to get tested. The best is a blood test that shows directly whether insulin level is normal or elevated. I usually send my patients for this test whenever there is a good reason for it (as the test is not cheap).

Another test is called the glucose tolerance test, which measures and compares the changes in blood glucose before and every half-hour after drinking a liquid sugar solution. It takes 3 hours. Blood glucose changes can indirectly establish the probability of hyperinsulinemia.

Many people with hyperinsulinemia have normal fasting glucose values (after 12 hours of not eating), which is why the common fasting blood glucose test doesn't work in the case of hyperinsulinemia.

People under constant stress are prone to developing hyperinsulinemia and overweight because stress hormones counter-regulate insulin, strengthening insulin resistance.

Among the factors that affect the glycemic index of foods are:

✦ Structure of starches in the food: slowly absorbed versus quickly absorbed.

✦ Kind of cooking: the more carbohydrates swell during cooking, the higher the glycemic index.

✦ Presence of dietary fibers: lowers the glycemic index.

✦ Form of carbohydrates: rolled, ground, or mashed carbohydrates have a higher glycemic index; those that have not been refined and maintain their protective coat have a lower index.

✦ Presence of fat: lowers the glycemic index but at the cost of many more calories.

For example, the glycemic index for baked potatoes (containing quickly absorbed starch) is 121, whereas Italian pasta made of durum hard wheat (containing a slowly absorbed starch), has the glycemic index 53. Whole-wheat bread, which contains bran (dietary fiber), has a lower glycemic index than white bread. White rice (short-grain), containing quickly absorbed starch, has a higher glycemic index (83) than long-grain basmati rice, containing slowly absorbed starch (68), and both have a lower glycemic index than white bread. Pasta, legumes, and various grains, containing both fiber and slowly absorbed starch, have lower glycemic indexes than white bread.

This does not mean that you can't occasionally eat potatoes or white rice, but on a daily basis, you would do better to choose foods with a lower glycemic index.

Protein foods, like meat, fish, eggs, and dairy products, contain almost no carbohydrates and do not significantly raise the blood glucose level. This is why so many popular diet programs focus on them. However, the glycemic index does not make up the whole picture. For example, proteins cause serotonin levels to decrease, and this has unwanted side effects like low moods (and even depression), irritability, restless sleep, concentration problems, cravings for sweets, and so forth. In addition, many protein-rich foods are also rich in fat and have very high caloric values. Together, this does not make for a healthy diet and prevents people from adhering to it for long.

The glycemic index is an excellent tool for selecting foods, especially among otherwise similar foods, in a more balanced and sensible manner, and its use reinforces the fact that in order to lose weight, you do not have to depend on counting calories.

Not only do snacks such as peanuts, jams, chocolate, chips, popcorn, and candy bars have a large number of calories, they also have a high glycemic index.

One word of caution. The glycemic index is not a precise measure and the value of a particular food will vary when it is combined with other foods.

MEASURES—NOT THE FULL PICTURE

Measuring the properties of food, such as calories, fat, carbohydrates and protein, plus glycemic index and glycemic load, are all important. However, they do not comprise the whole picture when it comes to dieting, losing weight and retaining your new weight. Though they are difficult to measure, the following may be at least as important:

+ How satisfying and filling your food choices are.

+ How long you remain satisfied after eating.

+ To what extent a food choice raises your serotonin.

+ Taste.

(continued on page 64)

PICKING YOUR CARBS

✦ ✦ ✦

Use this at-a-glance chart when selecting bread and other carbohydrates. The low-to-high range refers to how the foods score on the glycemic index. Low is always your best choice.

Best (LOW)	Good (MEDIUM)	Avoid (HIGH)
Pumpernickel bread	Rye bread	White bread, baguette
Rye bread with fiber	Whole-wheat bread	
Bread with a high fiber content		
Bran cereal	Muesli	Cornflakes
Oatmeal	Whole-wheat cookies	Cheerios
Cherries, apples, pears	Bananas, pineapples	Watermelons
Legumes (peas, broad beans, kidney beans, lentils, and soy beans)	Basmati rice	White rice
Pasta from durum wheat	Corn	Potatoes, mashed potatoes
Groats (oats, buck-wheat, pearl barley, wheat germ)	Sweet potatoes	
Nonsugar dairy products (can be artificially sweetened)	Ice cream	White and brown sugar, honey
Various kinds of vegetables	Carrots, beets	

GLYCEMIC INDEX: FOOD CHOICES AT A GLANCE

✦ ✦ ✦

The glycemic index plays an important role in *The Bread for Life Diet* because controlling insulin is one of the strategies that contribute to weight loss. The index is a generalized value of individual foods in comparison to white bread, which has a value of 100. Foods below 100 are insulin friendly; those above raise insulin accordingly. This should only be used as a general guide, as food pairings can affect an individual food's glycemic index value.

Food	Glycemic Index	Food	Glycemic Index
FRUITS		**LEGUMES**	
Cherries	32	Soy beans (dried/canned)	20
Grapefruit	36	Lentils (dried)	36
Apple	54	Kidney beans (dried)	43
Plum	55	Chick-peas (dried)	47
Peach	60	Green peas (dried)	50
Orange	63	Chick-peas (canned)	60
Grapes	66	Green peas (canned)	65
Pear	68	Baked beans (canned)	70
Banana	77	Kidney beans (canned)	74
Apricot	82	Lentils (canned)	74
Raisins	91		
Pineapple	94		
Watermelon	103		
Dates	142		

Food	Glycemic Index	Food	Glycemic Index
ROOT VEGETABLES		**BREAKFAST CEREALS**	
Sweet potato	70	Bran cereal	70
French fries	107	Oatmeal	89
Potato (baked)	121	Muesli	96
Potatoes (instant)	120	Cheerios	106
		Puffed wheat	110
BREAD		Cornflakes	119
Oat	68	Puffed rice	132
Pumpernickel	68		
Rye (light/dark)	89	**PASTA**	
Rye (crispbread)	95	Spaghetti (various)	58-77
White	100	Macaroni (durum wheat)	64
White flour bagel	103	Italian pasta (durum)	53
Whole-grain (various)	68-88	Rice Pasta	131
GRAINS		**SNACKS**	
Barley	36	Potato chips	77
Bulgur	65	Corn chips	99
Basmati rice	68	Doughnut	108
Buckwheat	78		
Sweet corn	78	**DAIRY PRODUCTS**	
Brown rice	79	Whole or skim milk	44
Popcorn	79	Yogurt	52
White rice	83	Ice cream	69
Rice cakes	117		

+ Effort involved in preparing the food.

+ Accessibility and cost of the food.

+How long you can maintain the diet without breaking it.

You can plainly see how bread, for one, excels in all of these areas and why it is the focus of *The Bread for Life Diet*. Nothing in life is really all good or all bad, all black or all white. There are trade-offs, and bread is one of the best trade-offs you can make. Its glycemic index/load and caloric value are not the lowest, but they are low enough that you can eat small amounts of it often enough to feel satisfied, for a long time and keep serotonin and your mood elevated.

Other options require you to eat a lot more (which means more calories!) to feel satisfied, or to eat foods (like protein) that lower serotonin levels, leaving you hungry and cranky. Yes, bread is one exception to the rule that the lower the glycemic index and caloric value, the better.

Another exception is fruit. In spite of having low glycemic index values, they can be fattening, so their consumption is limited on *The Bread for Life Diet*. However, when you have a choice between different types of breads and fruits, it's still better to select the ones with the lower glycemic index.

SUGAR IS NOT ESSENTIAL

I am often asked whether abstaining from sugar can be harmful, and the answer is: absolutely not! First of all, every carbohydrate turns into glucose during the digestive process, so any diet containing carbohydrates will provide enough glucose to keep the body functioning. Second, sugar is not a necessary source of nutrition for your body. Actually sugars are often called "empty calories." Until the sixteenth century, sugar wasn't commonly used at all in the Western world. Because of its price, only the wealthy could afford it, and even they used it only as a rare treat. Even after major geographic discoveries enabled the widespread distribution of sugar cane, sugar was still considered a luxury. Only after 1812, when sugar was produced from the sugar beet for the first time, did processed sugar become cheaper, and therefore a more common commodity.

Statistics show that in spite of all-out war against worldwide obesity, the average global consumption of sugar is going up. I hope the readers of my book can help buck this trend.

THE BREAD FOR LIFE DIET is based on understanding the central role insulin plays in weight gain and on the smart use of the glycemic index in making daily food choices. In addition to weight loss, *The Bread for Life Diet* has other significant benefits: It helps reduce blood sugar, insulin, fat, and cholesterol levels, and lowers blood pressure, thereby preventing the development of diabetes and heart disease.

6

Who This Diet Can Help

The Bread for Life Diet is a nutritious, well-balanced, easy-to-use weight-loss program. It has also been found to promote good health and reduce some of the risk factors that contribute to certain diseases. To me, this is much more than a fringe benefit. It is a gift of good health.

Though designed to help overweight people reduce their weight easily and healthily, *The Bread for Life Diet* is also a sensible eating plan for normal-weight people who want to eat healthfully.

This diet can work for anyone, with the possible exception of people who dislike bread and carbohydrate-rich foods. If you are overweight, have any risk factors for heart disease or diabetes, or are being treated for any medical condition, you should consult a physician before starting this program.

HAVE A HEALTH PROBLEM?

The Bread for Life Diet can be beneficial for the following:

+ People with heart disease.

+ Those who are at a high risk for heart disease.

+ People with high blood pressure.

+ People with type 2 diabetes.

+ People diagnosed with hypoglycemia.

+ People with high blood cholesterol.

+ People with high triglyceride levels.

+ Women who suffer from premenstrual syndrome.

+ People who suffer from chronic headaches.

+ People with depression, including those who take antidepressants.

+ People with chronic constipation.

+ People suffering from heartburn or acid reflux.

+ People under stress.

The principles of *The Bread for Life Diet* are suitable also for the following, but with certain adjustments. Again, consult with your physician or a registered dietitian first.

+ Children, adolescents, and pregnant or lactating women need to add dairy and low-fat meat products and make sure they are getting an adequate amount of calories as determined by their physicians or registered dietitians.

+ People with celiac disease (who cannot tolerate wheat products) need to replace bread and wheat products with rice and rice products, corn, potatoes, and gluten-free products.

Heart Disease

The healthy foods featured in the diet have been found to help alleviate the common risk factors for heart disease: diabetes, hyperinsulinemia, high cholesterol and/or triglyceride levels, high blood pressure, and excess weight. In addition, a high complex carbohydrate diet helps reduce the level of a special blood protein, C-reactive protein (CRP), which is a marker of inflammation. CRP is believed to be an important risk factor for heart disease.

High Blood Pressure

The major components of *The Bread for Life Diet*—complex carbohydrates, a relatively large volume of liquids, small frequent meals, dietary fiber, vegetable oils, and low-salt content—all jointly contribute to reducing blood pressure.

Diabetes

Although there is a widely held belief that people with diabetes should avoid bread and other carbohydrates, *The Bread for Life Diet* is beneficial for diabetic conditions for the following reasons:

+ *Complex* carbohydrates with a low glycemic index are necessary for maintaining balanced blood glucose and insulin levels.

+ Small meals, eaten every 3 to 4 hours, prevent blood glucose and insulin levels from rising.

- The diet substantially decreases the craving for sweets that is characteristic of most diabetics, thus helping them maintain lower blood glucose and insulin levels.

- *Complex* carbohydrates, including vegetables, are rich in vitamins and minerals, which are very important to those with diabetes.

- *Complex* carbohydrates, including vegetables, are rich in dietary fiber, also important to lowering blood glucose and insulin levels.

- The diet may postpone or even prevent the development of diabetes in prediabetic people.

The most recent recommendation of the American Diabetes Association is a diet comprised of 50 to 65 percent complex carbohydrates having a low glycemic index. This is fully consistent with *The Bread for Life Diet*.

Hypoglycemia

The Bread for Life Diet can help reduce the symptoms of hypoglycemia, a condition in which blood sugar levels drop drastically. Eating small meals high in complex carbohydrates and avoiding sweets prevent insulin levels from rising and glucose levels from dropping too much, keeping them relatively stable.

High Blood Cholesterol

Significant factors in reducing blood cholesterol level include:

- Actively consuming monounsaturated vegetable fats, such as olive and canola oil, which are the fat of choice on this diet.

- Severely limiting consumption of saturated fats.

✦ Actively consuming *complex* carbohydrates and vegetables containing dietary fiber necessary for lowering cholesterol levels.

High Triglyceride

Big rich meals, lots of sugar, and high fat intake make blood triglyceride levels go up. *The Bread for Life Diet* limits sugars and fats and recommends small meals, a potent tool for decreasing the triglyceride levels in the blood.

Premenstrual Syndrome

Because it emphasizes the consumption of *complex* carbohydrates, *The Bread for Life Diet* helps reduce tension, nervousness, and irritability, and its frequent small meals help prevent cravings. It is the perfect diet for premenstrual syndrome.

Headaches

Among the reasons for headaches are: lack of liquids (which causes chronic dehydration), hunger (caused by skipping meals), and a change in serotonin levels. The high complex carbohydrate content in *The Bread for Life Diet,* together with a large amount of liquids and small frequent meals, help relieve or prevent headaches.

Depression

Foods that are high in *complex* carbohydrates raise the level of serotonin, a neurotransmitter responsible for good moods and a general feeling of well-being, among other things. Actually, antidepressant drugs work in a similar way. Evidence suggests that a diet high in complex carbohydrates can strengthen the influence of antidepressant drugs.

Chronic Constipation

The Bread for Life Diet contains lots of fiber-rich vegetables and *complex* carbohydrates and encourages drinking 6 to 9 glasses of liquids a day, at a minimum. Consuming substantial amounts of fiber and liquids, together with small, frequent meals, is the best way to fight constipation.

Heartburn and Acid Reflux

Small, frequent *complex* carbohydrate meals do miracles in alleviating, sometimes even eliminating, heartburn attacks.

Stress

People who are under a lot of stress can benefit from *The Bread for Life Diet* because frequent meals rich in *complex* carbohydrates raise the serotonin level, which helps reduce tension and improve moods. It can be especially useful for helping people deal with their challenges, from students preparing for exams to top executives facing complex business challenges.

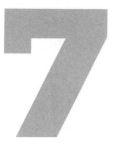

7

The Bread for Life Diet

Perhaps you have been on a diet before—likely several different kinds and with a varied mix of results. It's also likely that you know a lot about dieting and are familiar with many different diets. Since you're reading this book, I'm assuming that none of those diets worked for you, at least not in the long term. There may have been a good reason why they didn't work. For a diet to be successful, it has to offer the right tools.

No matter how many times we say, "I'll start counting calories tomorrow," "I won't eat anything sweet," or "I'll never touch bread again," we're doomed to fail because we aren't using an approach that will enable us to eat sensibly and lose weight.

The Bread for Life Diet provides the right tools with a practical, easy-to-follow menu that offers great-tasting foods and doesn't leave you hungry. *The Bread for Life Diet* allows you to choose from a wide variety of foods to suit your personal preferences, tastes, and lifestyle. It allows you to eat out in restaurants, at social gatherings, and even on vacation, because the wide choice of foods allowed makes it possible to find suitable dishes on most menus. Unbelievable as it may sound, *The Bread for Life Diet* helps stop the craving for sweets that can add too many calories to your daily total. In other words, this diet is proof that it is possible to overcome the challenges of weight loss while loving every minute!

Rest assured, this is not a fad diet. It is based on all of the scientific, physiological, and behavioral principles presented in this book:

+ The effect of serotonin on hunger and moods.

+ The effect of insulin on weight gain.

+ The effect of eating a wide variety of foods.

+ The glycemic index.

+ Energy balance.

+ Physical activity.

Plus three additional principles that you are sure to like:

+ No calorie counting.

+ No going hungry.

+ Balanced nutrition using all the food groups necessary for good health.

PRINCIPLES OF THE BREAD FOR LIFE DIET

The Bread for Life Diet is based on sound and proven principles that lead to weight loss, provide optimal nutrition, and promote good health.

These are those principles:

1. Eat Plenty of Bread and Other Complex Carbohydrates

The Bread for Life Diet is based on eating *complex* carbohydrates because they raise your serotonin level and provide a feeling of fullness and tranquility, help keep you alert, improve your mood, and allow you to function and perform at your peak. The type of carbohydrates in this program is important because it can affect the rate at which you will lose weight.

2. Eat Frequently

Eating *complex* carbohydrates every 3 to 4 hours prevents a drop in your serotonin level and eliminates the biological stumbling blocks that get in the way of dieting—hunger pangs, drowsiness, fatigue, a strong craving for sweet foods, irritability, bad moods, and restlessness, any of which can drive you to the refrigerator or cookie jar.

3. Never Skip a Meal

When you eat all your meals, you prevent a drop in blood sugar and serotonin levels, consequently reducing the strong desire and temptation to eat too much or to eat sweet foods because you never feel hungry.

Eating the "wrong" (simple) carbohydrates, such as sugar, causes insulin to soar, which contributes to faster weight gain. On *The Bread for Life Diet*, only complex carbohydrates are recommended. You select among foods containing carbohydrates according to their glycemic index. Foods with a low glycemic index help prevent a dramatic increase in blood sugar and insulin levels, thereby promoting weight loss.

4. Make Meals Small

Keeping meals small and spreading them throughout the day helps keep your serotonin level high, while insulin secretion stays relatively low. The result is that you feel full. It also encourages your body to burn energy.

Many of my patients, after being on *The Bread for Life Diet* for some time, say that when they eat an ordinary large meal with lots of meat and lots of carbohydrates, they feel heavy, full, and sleepy afterward. They wonder how they were able to eat that way for so many years.

5. Drink Plenty of Fluids

Your body is approximately 60 percent water, and fluids are important for its metabolism. All the body's chemistry occurs in water "media"—blood, lymph, cerebrospinal liquid, and so on. No less important is the fact that drinking enough liquid helps you feel more full, prevents dehydration, and generally improves the way you feel.

6. Do Some Physical Activity

The Bread for Life Diet goes hand-in-hand with physical exercise. Activities like walking or riding a bike burn off extra calories; lower lipid, sugar, and insulin levels in the blood; accelerate metabolism; increase the fat-burning process; and improve mood.

7. Take the Right Supplements

Multi-vitamin and calcium supplements are recommended for men and women and will complement your overall nourishment.

8. Take Time-Outs

Taking a "food break" gives you the chance to focus on yourself, even if it's just for a short while, and make the most of the cephalic stage of eating. Eating small, frequent meals offers the perfect opportunity for taking a time out. And, if you take time-outs during your busiest hours, it may help relieve your stress levels too!

9. Remember, the Rules Are Flexible

The Bread for Life Diet recognizes that the principle of "all or nothing" is neither effective nor supportive for people trying to lose weight. Even if you occasionally eat items that are not allowed, you can still get back on track easily and continue to lose weight. The diet makes allowances for mistakes and setbacks. Nothing happens if you have a bad eating day. You just get back on the diet the next day. There is no reason to ever give up and gain the weight you lost back.

A HEALTH BONUS

The results of *The Bread for Life Diet*, as demonstrated by thousands of people, are:

- ✦ Successful weight loss
- ✦ Loss in abdominal fat
- ✦ Decrease in total and "bad" cholesterol
- ✦ Drop in triglyceride levels
- ✦ Lower blood pressure
- ✦ Improvement in blood sugar levels
- ✦ Better insulin control
- ✦ More vitality
- ✦ Improved concentration
- ✦ Fewer mood swings
- ✦ Better sleep
- ✦ Improved self-image

HIGHLIGHTS OF THE BREAD FOR LIFE DIET

There are three major categories of food on *The Bread for Life Diet*:

+ Recommended, unlimited (e.g., vegetables)

+ Recommended, limited (e.g., bread, fruits)

+ Not recommended (e.g., processed foods, high-fat red meat, fats, sweets)

The diet has two stages:

Stage One is more rigorous and lasts up to 2 weeks. This stage is designed to produce faster weight loss and is based mainly on eating slices of bread with thin spreads.

Stage Two includes more food choices, lasts for an unlimited time (even for a lifetime), incorporates many substitutes for bread slices, and results in a more moderate rate of weight loss. It is also the model for weight maintenance. If pounds start to creep back on, return to Stage One.

+ There is no classification of major meals versus minor meals, or breakfast/lunch/dinner versus 10-o'clock or 5-o'clock breaks. You eat every 3 to 4 hours throughout all waking hours.

+ Eat the first meal 1 to 3 hours after you wake up, and eat the last meal 1 to 2 hours before you go to sleep.

+ Eat *before* you get hungry so you do not find yourself eating more than the recommended amount.

- Light (not white) bread is recommended over regular bread because it allows you to eat twice as many slices, which contributes to the feeling of satiety.

- You can eat bread a single slice at a time or as a 2-slice sandwich.

- You can enhance your bread or sandwich with any amount of the unlimited foods (e.g., vegetables) and/or a thin layer/slice of limited foods (e.g., fat-free mayonnaise, turkey, tuna).

- Women should drink at least seven or eight, and men eight or nine, 8-ounce glasses of water or sugar-free, nonalcoholic beverages each day, tea and coffee included.

- When you eat, concentrate on the food, not on anything else like TV, a newspaper, or a book.

- Prior to every meal, you have a moment of choice. There may be times you will choose foods that aren't recommended or more than the recommended amounts. This implies nothing about your next choice. If you "break" the diet with an unrecommended choice, nothing bad happens. At your next meal, just pick up where you left off.

THE TWO STAGES OF THE BREAD FOR LIFE DIET

Stage One promotes fast weight loss and helps break some of the nasty habits that result in overeating and overweight. However, any diet that limits food variety has a limit to how much a person can take. This is mainly why I recommend it for about a week, and definitely no more than 2 weeks, at a time. Though it is nutritionally balanced, it is not intended for long-term use. It is, however, a plan you can go back to whenever you feel your diet is stalled or you notice that you are beginning to gain a few pounds.

Stage One is also designed to help get your insulin and serotonin levels under control. During Stage One, your sugar and insulin levels will start to improve, your serotonin level will stabilize, and you will begin to experience a sense of enjoyment—a wonderful feeling that will encourage you to continue with the diet. The diet works to "straighten out" these two body substances.

People with type 2 diabetes or with prediabetes, in rare cases, may experience a drop in blood glucose during this transitional stage. This can present itself as a sudden weakness or dizziness. This is no cause for alarm, it is a sign that your insulin is beginning to stabilize and work better. If it happens, however, be sure to do the following:

+ Consult your doctor. If you are on diabetic drugs, your doctor may want to decrease the dosage or change the type of drug you take. *Do not cut back on your medication on your own!*

+ Eat a small *complex* carbohydrate meal every 3 or even 2 hours. *Do not skip meals!*

+ Have with you a piece of fruit, a cracker, or even a piece of candy to eat as soon as you begin to feel a symptom coming on. If you do not miss a meal, however, this should not be necessary.

+ Drink enough liquids; dehydration can lead to similar symptoms. Women should drink seven to eight 8-ounce glasses a day and men should drink eight to nine glasses a day.

Remember that these symptoms are usually signs of improvement and they will go away as your insulin stabilizes.

Stage Two is much more relaxed because it is intended for the long haul and is meant to be the basis of an eating style you can follow for the rest of your life. Stage Two has so much variety, freedom, and choice that making it a way of life really isn't difficult. If your discipline becomes a bit lax, or if you happen to reach a weight-loss plateau, you can always return to Stage One for 3 to 10 days to speed up your weight loss, and then return to Stage Two.

GENERAL GUIDELINES FOR STAGES ONE AND TWO

The following guidelines apply to both Stage One and Stage Two. They explain the importance of eating frequent meals and how to include bread, vegetables, meats, dairy products, and other foods in your daily eating plan. A sample day and some sample meals for both stages are included as well.

One of the charms of *The Bread for Life Diet* is its simplicity. Foods are easy to prepare. However, there are people who love to experiment with new diet recipes, so I offer some of my favorites in the Bread for Life Recipes chapter on page 187.

1. Bread Every Day

True to its name, *The Bread for Life Diet* is based on eating bread (or its substitutes) every day—up to 16 slices of *light* bread a day for a man or up to 12 slices for a woman.

By *light* bread I mean breads that are about 35 to 45 calories per slice as opposed to regular bread, which has 80 or more calories per slice. Both Arnold and Pepperidge Farm are examples of brands that make light whole-grain breads in this calorie range.

If you choose regular bread instead of light, you will have to cut the amount of bread you eat in half. Note that there are gourmet breads, such as those containing nuts or raisins, that may well exceed 90 calories per slice. These are not recommended for everyday use but they are not forbidden. Just make sure to stay within your daily bread quota. Read the

SLICING THE SUBSTITUTES

When I refer to a slice of bread, I am referring to a slice of *light*, whole-grain (not white) bread in the range of 35 to 45 calories. Refer to this chart when choosing bread or a bread substitute, such as an English muffin or a bagel. If a slice of bread contains 120 calories, it is equivalent to three slices of light bread. Here are some equivalents for common items found in the supermarket:

- ✦ Pita bread = 4 slices of light bread
- ✦ 8-inch tortilla = 4 slices of light bread
- ✦ 10-inch tortilla = 6 slices of light bread
- ✦ Taco shell = 1 1/2 slices of light bread
- ✦ Hot dog roll = 3 slices of light bread
- ✦ Small hamburger bun = 3 slices of light bread
- ✦ Wrap = 3 slices of light bread
- ✦ Small bagel = 4 slices of light bread

label on the bread (and on all foods) carefully with special attention to the serving size (some breads list the serving size as one slice and others list it as two slices) and check out the number of calories per slice.

When choosing bread, it is important to choose whole-grain bread because its glycemic index is lower than that of white bread. You can eat a slice of white bread occasionally, but whole-grain bread should be your bread of choice for everyday use. Finding one or two kinds of bread you like is important, because I want you to enjoy your food and feel good about the diet and it will help you maintain the diet indefinitely.

Many people prefer European-style breads, which are a good choice because they often feature whole-grain, sprouted, or cracked wheat at the top of the ingredient lists. Not only are these the right breads for keeping your serotonin high, they are also high on the satisfaction scale and are usually healthy.

Stay away from bread that lists refined wheat white flour or corn syrup at or near the top of the list. These are all ingredients that tempt insulin. Ingredients are listed by the amount present in the food, starting with the greatest. If sugar is in the list, especially near the top, stay away from it.

WHAT'S LIGHT, WHAT'S NOT

Even though you don't need to count calories on *The Bread for Life Diet*, you should know the difference between regular products and products marked "light," "low-calorie," "low-fat," and "fat-free." Generally speaking, products with 1.4 or fewer grams of fat per ounce are okay, even though some fats are healthier than others. Products marked "low-fat" and "fat-free" are fine as long as they don't contain sugar. Sugar can be listed on nutrition labels under many different names, including glucose, grape sugar, fructose, and corn syrup.

Once you know how to interpret nutrition labels, you can expand your menu to include foods you love that are not specifically mentioned in this book. Just remember that many "light" products may be lighter than their "regular" counterparts, but still quite fattening and not light enough for *The Bread for Life Diet*.

2. Sandwich Variety

What can you spread and put on your bread? You can have a single *thin* layer of just about *anything* except sweet spreads. The exceptions include butter and regular (hard) margarine. Butter is almost 100 percent saturated fat and most margarines contain manufactured trans-fatty acids, reason enough to avoid them from a health standpoint. Here are some examples of what you can spread on your bread:

+ Mustard of your choice.

+ Ketchup, low-fat or fat-free mayonnaise, low-fat or fat-free salad dressing, or butter substitute made of vegetable oils that do not contain trans-fatty acids.

+ Cheese spread, especially fat-free and light cheese (cheese with a fat content less than 5 percent or 1.4 grams per ounce).

+ Hummus

+ Tahini

+ Mashed avocados

+ Salsa

+ Garlic paste

+ Anchovy

+ Sugar-free peanut butter

+ Icra (fish-based spread)

+ Caviar

+ Eggplant in tahini or in mayonnaise

- Soy spreads

- Natural tofu

- Canned or smoked tuna or sardines (squeeze out all the oil)

- A slice of smoked fish, like salmon

- A thin slice of any lean, low-fat meat, such as chicken or turkey

- Occasionally, you can put a slice of regular American or Swiss cheese on your sandwich, although low-fat cheese is better.

- If you really crave something sweet, you can put a small amount of sugar-free jam on your bread. Keep in mind, though, that although it does not have added sugar, it still contains a high concentration of fructose, with all associated consequences, if you eat too much.

3. Thin Is In—for Spreads

Even more important than what you put on your bread is how much you put on. Thinness is key. The spread must be very thin. In other words, you should eat *bread with a spread*, and not *a spread with bread*. It is also important that the sandwich contain only one type of spread, not two or three as you may be accustomed to. More might be a little bit tastier, but it is much more fattening.

The purpose of the spread is to satisfy your sense of taste. If you keep in mind that a teaspoon of low-fat cream cheese or cottage cheese, for example, tastes exactly the same as a whole container, you'll learn to spread an amount that allows you to lose weight with greater ease and efficiency and you won't miss out on flavor. A little really does go a long way.

One of my patients said to me: "I began to recognize the wonderful taste of bread, which I had forgotten because I used to put on so much dressing it covered up the taste of the bread. Now I taste the bread and the spread just adds to its flavor. I make the same sandwiches for my children as I do for myself, and they like them! They don't bring them back from school untouched."

4. Pile on the Vegetables

Once you've put spread on your bread, add vegetables in unlimited amounts. Pile on the lettuce, tomatoes, cucumbers, sprouts, carrots, onions, and whatever else you want in a sandwich. Or you can have a side salad, a serving of cooked vegetables, or a cup of vegetable soup to go with your sandwich. Besides being really quite a bit to eat, very filling and easy to prepare, it's also healthy!

One of my patients began the diet declaring that she hated vegetables, and ended up 25 pounds lighter with a passion for eating green beans cooked in the microwave. This just demonstrates that everything is a matter of making a decision and sticking to it until it becomes a habit.

The most noteworthy advantage of eating vegetables is the small amount of calories they contain and their very low rating on the glycemic index. In other words, they do not significantly increase sugar and insulin levels, and they help you to feel full. In addition, they are high in fiber, which is important for your satiety and general health, and they help keep the digestive system running smoothly. Best of all, you can eat all the vegetables you want, except for potatoes, sweet potatoes, corn and legumes.

In addition to being tasty and filling, vegetables are also rich in vitamins and minerals. For example, orange-colored and dark green vegetables (such as carrots, pumpkin, spinach, and peppers) contain the antioxidant beta-carotene, which has been found to guard against heart disease and cancer. Peppers, tomatoes, cabbage, and onions contain vitamin C, another antioxidant with numerous health and healing properties. Tomatoes, green beans, and parsley contain the mineral potassium, which is essential to keeping electrolytes in balance. Vegetables also contain phytochemicals, which are not vitamins but have their own special health-promoting properties. And the list goes on.

Color is often the key to a vegetable's healthfulness. The more variety in color you put on your plate, the healthier your meal will be.

For the most part, all vegetables (except for potatoes, sweet potatoes, and corn) are considered "free" foods on this diet. Take advantage of all the different types of each vegetable available, too. You may have unlimited amounts of the following (including all varieties of each):

+ Artichokes

+ Asparagus

+ Beets

+ Carrots

+ Celery

+ Cruciferous, or cabbage-family, vegetables (including broccoli, cauliflower, and Brussels sprouts)

+ Cucumbers

+ Eggplant

+ Fresh herbs

+ Garlic

+ Lettuce

+ Mushrooms, all varieties

+ Onions

+ Peppers(sweet and hot)

+ Pumpkin

+ Radishes

+ Spinach

+ Sprouts

+ Squash

+ String beans

+ Tomatoes (including tomato puree)

+ Turnips

+ Zucchini

VEGETABLES IN NAME ONLY

Potatoes, sweet potatoes, corn, and legumes are not included in the "unlimited" list because of their high starch content. They are allowed, however, as a bread substitute.

Pickled vegetables are also allowed in unlimited quantities. This, however, does not apply to people who must follow a salt-restricted diet.

5. Preparation Makes a Difference

You can prepare vegetables any way you like—fresh, boiled, grilled, steamed, stir-fried in a small amount of canola or olive oil, and in a vegetable soup. Keep in mind that cooking to some extent robs vegetables of some of their nutritional value, so try to use quicker ways of cooking that require high heat. When cooking vegetables in water, do not add them until the water reaches the boiling point. Because some of the nutrients leach into the water, you can save the water for making a soup. It will help spike its nutrient value.

You can also prepare vegetables by steaming them using a perforated pot insert that prevents the food from contacting the water. It will be more healthful if you can become accustomed to having your veggies a little *al dente* rather than cook them down to a purée.

Stir-frying is another healthful and flavorful way of preparing vegetables. Even though you add some oil (preferably olive or canola), their nutrients are mostly preserved.

Another way to preserve vitamins and minerals is to avoid cutting the vegetables before eating or cooking them. Cutting causes a significant loss in nutrient content, due to oxidation. The smaller the pieces, the greater the loss. When possible, eat vegetables whole or cut the pieces as large as possible. If you must chop, do so just before adding them to a recipe. If you prefer your salad finely chopped, eat and enjoy, but know that you're losing some nutrients. When possible, do not remove the skin from your vegetables because it contains dietary fiber, phytochemicals, vitamins, and minerals.

Vegetables also lose some of their vitamins if they are stored unfrozen for a long time, especially if they are exposed to moisture and different temperatures. Frozen vegetables actually have more nutritional value than fresh vegetables that have been stored improperly or for a long period of time.

A CURE FOR VEGETABLE AVOIDERS

There are people who claim they hate vegetables but it usually turns out that the aversion is more to the way the vegetables are prepared rather than to the vegetables themselves. One technique that may help turn you on to vegetables is adding a tablespoon or two of instant soup or broth mix to the water or liquid when cooking vegetable dishes. The reason they improve flavor is because most of these products contain monosodium glutamate (MSG). People who must follow a salt-restricted diet should not overuse these products.

For years, we had been warned to avoid MSG, which is common in Chinese food and a variety of ready-to-eat dishes. Now, however, it is generally agreed that eating MSG in moderation does not have a harmful effect on most people. There is no reason to avoid using it unless you are oversensitive to it and develop symptoms such as headaches, facial flushing, chest pressure or pain, and dizziness (so-called "Chinese restaurant syndrome").

Monosodium glutamate is naturally found in breast milk, tomatoes, mushrooms, meat, processed cheeses, and other foods.

Though the reaction to vegetables differs from one person to the next, people bothered by gas after eating certain vegetables will prefer cooked vegetables. Vegetables known to cause gas are cabbage, cauliflower, broccoli, Brussels sprouts, radishes, onions, and various kinds of peppers.

6. Fruit in Moderation

Most people consider fruit to be healthful food and it is—to a degree. Fruit is good for you because it contains vitamins, minerals, phytochemicals, and dietary fiber. (As with vegetables, avoid peeling or cutting fruit whenever possible to protect the nutrient and fiber content.) However, most of us tend to ignore its sugar content.

People think that fruit sugar, known as fructose, is okay because it is natural. Let me remind you that table sugar is also natural; it comes from the sugar beet, and meat fat is also completely natural. Even snake poison is natural. Natural doesn't automatically mean healthy. That's why the legitimacy of eating fruit can lead to eating excessive amounts, and this is where it crosses the line to unhealthy.

People often come to me and confess, with a clear conscience, that they do not eat candy, but they can polish off a bowl of fruit in one sitting. I've had people tell me they eat a couple of pounds of fruit a day—or more! Not a good idea if you care about your weight. Fruit gets its sweetness from a form of sugar called fructose, which has an advantage. It doesn't affect insulin as quickly as does white/brown table sugar. But eat too much and it acts just like any other sugar, causing a significant rise in blood glucose and triglyceride levels and, eventually, a rise in your weight, too. One theory suggests that fruit sugar converts into fat easily.

Because it is an overall nutritious food and because it can appease a sweet tooth, fruit is allowed on *The Bread for Life Diet*, but in moderation and in measured quantities. But just because you *can* eat fruit doesn't mean you *must* eat it. Still, it is always better to choose fruit over candy.

There is no need to be concerned that you'll miss out on certain nutrients if you avoid fruit. Rest assured, every nutrient that is present in fruits is present in vegetables, but without the sugar.

One serving of fruit is considered to be:

+ 1 apple

+ 2 or 3 apricots

+ 1 banana

+ 1 cup cherries

+ ½ grapefruit

+ Small bunch of grapes (preferably red)

+ 2 kiwifruits

+ 2 mandarin oranges

+ 1 nectarine

+ 1 orange

+ 2 passion fruits

+ 1 pear

+ 1 peach

+ 2 or 3 plums

+ 2 prickly pears

+ 1 cup strawberries

+ 1 slice of watermelon or honeydew melon

You can figure out where I am going with this. All fruits are permissible but you should use your judgment as to what serving to choose. Size is the key. Buy fruits that are medium- or even small-size. They might not look as appealing in a bowl on the table, but when you eat a piece, you'll be saving calories.

When selecting a serving of fruit, consider its glycemic index. Do not eat more than one serving at a time so you do not raise the glucose and triglyceride levels in your blood too much. Eat fruit as a separate snack and not as a dessert. Finishing a meal with fruit adds sugar and, together with a full meal, can raise the insulin level higher than optimal. It is best to save fruit for between meals when you may feel you want something sweet.

Avoid drinking fruit juice and eating stewed fruit and fruit salads. All contain a high concentration of sugar. Even if no white or brown sugar has been added to them, they contain more sugar, have a much higher glycemic index, and contain considerably less vitamins and fiber than the fruit itself. A glass of juice has the equivalent of 5 to 6 teaspoons of sugar.

7. Meat, Poultry, and Fish Are Welcome

Protein in the form of meat, poultry, or fish is permitted three meals a week during Stage One and up to five times a week during Stage Two. Do not eat any bread or any other carbohydrates at the meat meal. As a side dish, use all kinds of vegetables in unlimited amounts (excluding potatoes, sweet potatoes, and corn). Also, on the days you choose to eat meat, poultry, or fish, women should reduce their daily quota of bread to six to eight slices and men to ten slices. Meat, poultry, and fish are encouraged because they are an important component of human nutrition. Animal food constitutes an excellent source of high-quality proteins, and supplies iron, zinc, vitamins B_{12}, B_6, and other nutrients. Animal food can be very rich in fat, however, most of which is saturated and should be avoided, as it raises blood cholesterol levels, adding to the risk of cardiovascular disease. So be sure to select lean meats.

Vegetarians can replace meat with soy dishes, soy flakes, or tofu. Rigorous vegetarians may have deficiencies in the nutrients that animal meats supply, especially iron and B12, and should discuss supplementation with their doctors or dietitians.

Recommended meats and poultry:

+ Chicken—all parts, with the skin and all visible fat removed

+ Turkey—all parts, with the skin and all visible fat removed

+ Beef and pork—cut from the hindquarter (such as filet, sirloin, tenderloin, round, rump, shank), with all visible fat removed

+ Ostrich

+ Veal filet or leg—with all visible fat removed.

+ Venison

Avoid:

+ Corned beef

+ Duck

+ Flank steak

+ Goose

+ Ground beef

+ Ham

+ Lamb

+ Porterhouse steak

+ Processed meats and sausages

+ Ribs

+ T-bone steak

Seafood and fish are excellent sources of protein, iron, and other nutrients. They are relatively lean and I highly recommend them. In principle, all fish and seafood are permitted, including lobster, scallops, and shrimp.

Cold-water ocean fish are especially healthy, because they contain omega-3 fatty acids, an oil known to help prevent certain diseases such as heart disease, cancer, inflammatory diseases, hypertension, and others. Types of fish that contain generous amounts of omega-3 are salmon, mackerel, tuna (though canned tuna is devoid of much of the protective oil), trout, cod, herring, sardines, hake, sole, and halibut. Scientific research has shown that people who eat these kinds of fish two to three times a week have, on average, a lower incidence of heart disease.

Meat, poultry, and fish can be eaten grilled, broiled, baked, roasted, sautéed with a small amount of oil, stir-fried in a wok, boiled, or quickly fried in a small amount of oil. It is preferable to use olive or canola oil.

Do not dredge or coat your meat, chicken, or fish with flour or bread-crumbs because carbohydrates like these absorb a lot of oil while frying, which adds fat and calories. Also, avoid meat sauces or gravies, which can contain a lot of fat. The best sauce for fish is lemon juice and a small amount of olive oil.

Be sure that all visible fat and chicken and turkey skin are removed before and/or after cooking. After frying, remove the remaining fat or oil by draining or blotting the food with absorbent paper towels. You can add herbs and spices in unlimited amounts.

When you have your meat meals, eat as much meat, poultry, or fish as you like (within reason—not the whole chicken!). You might want to reserve these meals for when you go out to a restaurant, dine at a friend's house, or on a weekend when you have more time to prepare meals.

8. No Bread with Protein Meals

This is not for the purpose of separating proteins and carbohydrates—a very popular theory on some diets, but not on *The Bread for Life Diet*. The only reason you don't eat bread with these meals is to keep the meal smaller and less diverse. Remember, the more diverse the meal, the more you eat. Large meals—a big steak and potatoes is a classic example—will raise your insulin level. This is exactly what you do not want to happen.

9. Eggs Any Style

You can eat three or four eggs a week, including the yolk, prepared any way you like, including fried in a small amount of oil (but not in butter or margarine). You can eat eggs with bread.

Eggs are highly nutritious. They have the highest protein value of any food and are high in other nutrients, such as vitamin B_{12}. Eggs are tasty, nutritious, cheap, and an easy meal solution. When eaten as a part of a low-saturated fat diet, eggs do not raise cholesterol levels, in spite of the fact that they do contain cholesterol. Today it is known that the blood cholesterol level is mostly influenced by saturated fat and not by pure cholesterol as found in eggs.

Adding unsaturated fat to the diet helps decrease the blood cholesterol level even more. In two ongoing large population studies at Harvard University, one involving nurses and the other physicians, research found that egg consumption is not related to cardiovascular risk, but saturated fat consumption is. I participated in an Israeli study in which we gave one to three eggs a day within a low-saturated-fat diet to people with moderately increased cholesterol levels for 9 weeks. There was no increase in the cholesterol levels in any of the participants.

So you can eat eggs three or four times a week even if you have high cholesterol, but on two conditions: Have your cholesteral monitored and follow my diet rigorously. Specifically, be sure to reduce your overall saturated fat consumption and increase your consumption of unsaturated fats, especially monounsaturated fats like olive oil and canola oil.

10. Dairy Products—only Unsugared and Low-Fat

Dairy products are permitted, but with limitations. On *The Bread for Life Diet*, milk is considered a food, not a drink. You can add low-fat milk (up to 2 percent fat) to your coffee or tea or drink it by itself, but do not exceed 8 ounces of milk a day, and the less the better. You can substitute soy milk (without sugar) for dairy milk.

Other dairy foods are permissible if they contain no more than 5 percent fat or 1.4 grams of fat per ounce (28 grams).

Select only cheeses—cottage cheese, soft cheeses, salty cheeses, or processed cheese—that meet this criterion. Be cautious when selecting yogurt or pudding. Many low-fat or fat-free products claim to be "light" or boast "0% fat" but make up the difference by adding lots of sugar. Read the labels and make sure that they are sweetened with artificial sweeteners, if at all.

Not recommended are butter, cream, whipped cream, and any cheese with a high fat content (over 5% fat). The reason is obvious: They are fattening and unhealthy.

11. Oils Are a Must

In spite of its caloric content, this is the steadfast rule concerning oils: You must consume 2 to 3 tablespoons (not teaspoons) of olive or canola oil a day. Even though oil is caloric, it is important to your health. Oils that are high in monounsaturated fats and low in saturated fats are an important component of a healthful diet because they contain the fatty acids that are essential for good health and help reduce bad (LDL) cholesterol levels while maintaining good (HDL) cholesterol levels.

A dietary bonus is that it makes the rest of the diet more enjoyable. It means you don't have to eat dry salads or salads with just vinegar. Olive and canola oils are also the recommended fats for frying, sautéing, and baking. Occasionally, especially in sauces, oil can be replaced by low-calorie mayonnaise, but it is not advisable to do so often.

Contrary to popular belief, quick frying over high heat does not harm the quality of the oil used. This holds true for oil used to fry eggs, onions, chicken, steak, or other protein foods, or to stir-fry vegetables.

A WORD ABOUT OLIVES

Olive oil comes from olives, and both are healthful, but they should not be considered equals when it comes to the diet. Olives are high in calories and people tend to eat several at a sitting rather than just a few. It is best to avoid them.

During Stage One, you should avoid olives. During Stage Two, you can have a few once in a while, possibly cut up and put into a sandwich. Ten olives are equivalent to 1 tablespoon of oil.

Deep-fat frying, however, and especially reusing leftover oil, damages the quality of oil because it causes it to oxidize. This is just something you should know, as you should not be eating deep-fried foods anyway!

Be cautious when sautéing in oil because certain foods absorb oil like a sponge. Eggplant is a perfect example. Sauté in a nonstick pan and use heat to help reduce the amount of oil needed. In some cases, you don't need to use oil at all. For example, an excellent way to fry onions without oil is simply to put the onions in a covered nonstick pan over high heat. This process cooks the onions in their own juices. The result is tasty, golden, crisp, and oil-free "fried" onions.

12. Some Fats Are Out

I do not recommend using any type of margarine, even though it is made from vegetable fat, except those that do not contain trans-fatty acids. Most margarines are made by hydrogenating vegetable oils to make them solid at room temperature, and they contain trans-fatty acids, which are currently under fire for being unhealthful. Research shows that they not only raise overall cholesterol levels, they lower the good (HDL) cholesterol.

There are, however, new brands of spreads made without trans fats such as Benecol and Take Control. Choose them instead and use as directed for any spread on the diet.

Hydrogenated fats are widely used in ready-to-eat foods, such as cakes, cookies, puff pastries, and so on. Read the labels to recognize and avoid them.

Fats that you should avoid on *The Bread for Life Diet* in addition to margarine include butter, animal fat, poultry skin, coconut oil, and date oil. Not only do they add calories but they contain saturated fat.

13. Eat All Day

Eating every 3 to 4 hours is key to the success of *The Bread for Life Diet* because it keeps insulin levels steady and serotonin levels regularly elevated.

EXTRA FAT FACTS

If you really want to know how low the fat is in a particular food, you need to look for products that contain no more than 5 percent fat by weight. You compute the fat percentage by multiplying the number of fat grams in a serving by 100 and dividing by the serving size. For example, if a product has 4 grams of fat per serving, and a serving size of 28 grams, 4 times 100 divided by 28 yields 14 percent. Do not confuse percentage of fat with percentage of Recommended Daily Value.

Choosing foods this way can become complicated , so I recommend just sticking to products that do not contain any type of sugar (not just "no sugar *added*," but also no honey, fructose, corn syrup, etc.) and are either "low-fat" or "fat-free." Double-check products marked "light": These are lighter in calories than their nonlight counterparts, but are usually not light enough for everyday use.

Eating frequently also guarantees that you won't be hungry. Not being hungry, however, is not a sign that you should skip a meal. Quite the opposite is true. By skipping meals, you will undo the diet and tempt all the biological reactions that contribute to weight gain.

I hear time and again from people that this is most problematic in the morning because they just can't face food first thing. That is okay as long as you eat your first meal within 1 to 3 hours after you wake up. If that means 9:00 or 10:00, even 11:00 (if you wake up late), that's okay. But do not wait until you are hungry. Once you eat your first meal, you must eat at 3- to 4-hour intervals throughout the day. Remember that the body burns off energy in response to a meal, whereas hunger makes the body hoard fat because it slows down metabolism.

Many people ask, "Do I really have to eat if I'm not hungry?" The answer is a definite *yes*. When you wait too long for the next meal, you will inevitably and suddenly become hungry, maybe even ravenous. By then it is too late to eat as planned, and there is a real chance your eating will get out of control. The slogan "You must eat to lose weight" is very appropriate here.

14. Eat at Night

You can eat late in the evening, depending on your sleeping habits. In any case, I don't want you to go to bed hungry, so always leave some spare food for the end of the evening—a slice of light bread with a small amount of spread; a cup of yogurt; a low-fat, low-calorie pudding; a small piece of fruits or half a glass of warm milk.

The once-held belief that you should stop eating in the early evening is most likely based on human behavior of ancient times when people would go to sleep at sunset and wake up at dawn. Since the waking hours of modern people have been significantly extended, we don't need to follow this ancient custom. It would be ridiculous for a person who is awake until 1:00 in the morning to stop eating at 6:00 in the evening. Moreover, a small meal approximately 45 minutes before going to bed will help you sleep more soundly.

There are also circumstances when a nighttime meal is essential, such as for people with diabetes, hypoglycemia, ulcers, and other health problems.

I have found that a nighttime meal also helps those with a snoring problem or sleep apnea. People with these conditions have reported that the diet helped ease their symptoms and even eliminate them. The first and foremost reason for this is due to the decrease in weight. However, I've noticed through my research that a small *complex* carbohydrate meal or half a glass of warm milk can help elevate serotonin, which contributes to a peaceful night's sleep.

15. Lots of Fluids

I recommend drinking plenty of fluids, for several reasons. A lack of fluids causes dehydration and dehydration slows down weight loss. Even if you don't feel thirsty, it does not mean you don't need fluid. That's why I recommend that women drink seven to eight 8-ounce glasses a day and men eight to nine glasses. When it is hot and humid, you should get even more. Just don't overdo it. Drinking more than 15 glasses a day under ordinary conditions is unnecessary, not recommended, and can even be harmful.

By fluids I do not mean you must be limited to water. You can have any nonsugared, nonalcoholic drink, such as mineral water, diet soda, seltzer water, tea, fruit juice (with artificial sweeteners), tomato juice, and other vegetable juices. Clear broth can count as a fluid, as opposed to soup with noodles or vegetables, which does not.

Beverages containing sugar, including flavored drinks, sodas, natural juices, sweetened juices, and reconstituted juices, are not recommended. Remember, a standard can (12 ounces) of any sugar-containing beverage or natural fruit juice can contain approximately 8 teaspoons of sugar!

16. Caffeine Is Okay

There are many myths regarding coffee and tea because of their caffeine content. Caffeine will not affect your success on *The Bread for Life Diet*.

Usually the only problem with drinking tea and coffee is that people add cream or milk and sugar or eat cake or cookies with it. Unless you are sensitive to the side effects of caffeine, you can drink as much coffee or tea as you want, as long as the total milk consumed per day does not exceed one glass a day (the less milk the better) and you use an artificial sweetener in place of sugar.

Regular black tea and green tea contain special substances called polyphenols that act like an anti-oxidant and help prevent heart disease and cancer. They may even help improve bone density. Recent research shows that tea and coffee have a favorable effect in prevention of type 2 diabetes. Coffee can make some people feel nervous, and it can prevent sleep or cause irregular heartbeats.

17. Artificial Sweeteners

If you prefer your beverages or food sweetened, using artificial sweeteners such as saccharine or aspartame is recommended. White and brown sugars and honey are not recommended for daily use if you want to lose weight. Health organizations in both the United States and Europe consider these products to be free of any harmful effects. The U.S. Food and Drug Administration (FDA) has even removed saccharine from the list of carcinogens, where it had been listed since the 1960s.

Some people don't like artificial sweeteners, claiming that they taste artificial and leave an after-taste. Artificial sweeteners may take some getting used to, but once you do, things get reversed. Suddenly it's sugar that tastes weird and leaves an after-taste! This is what happened to me—I didn't like artificial sweeteners at all at first. It also happened to almost all my clients who initially did not like artificial sweeteners. It is sure worth trying.

18. Go Light on Alcohol, If at All

Alcohol is not considered a drink on *The Bread for Life Diet* and does not count in your daily allotment of liquids. It is allowed, in limited quantity, for those who can't or do not want to do without.

The negatives of alcohol, in relationship to this diet, are that it is absorbed rapidly into the bloodstream and it contains 7 calories per gram (compared to 4 per gram in protein and carbohydrates and 9 in fat). These are calories devoid of any nutritional value.

Alcohol is only allowed in moderation during both stages of the diet. To make the most of it, choose red wine over all others because it contains substances that have been found to be beneficial to heart health. Women should drink with prudence because they have less of the enzyme dehydrogenase, which helps break down alcohol, so they do not metabolize alcohol as well as men. Another caution for women is that alcohol consumption has been linked to an increased risk of breast cancer.

19. Condiments Are Allowed

There are many allowable ingredients that you would not use as a bread spread but that can be used to flavor food or add to sauce recipes. Those allowed in unlimited amounts include:

+ Herbs
+ Lemon juice
+ Mushrooms

+ Soy sauce
+ Tomato juice/puree
+ Vinegars

In limited amounts, you may add:

+ Ketchup
+ Mayonnaise (low-fat or fat-free)
+ Vegetable oils (preferably canola or olive)

DON'T GO BELOW THE MINIMUM

+ Do not reduce your overall daily food intake below the recommended amounts.

+ Do not skip any meals.

+ On ordinary days, women eat at least 4 slices of regular bread or 8 slices of light bread and men eat at least 6 slices of regular bread or 12 slices of light bread.

+ On days when you eat meat or fish, women should eat at least 3 slices of regular bread or 6 slices of light bread, and men at least 5 slices of regular bread or 10 slices of light bread.

During Stage Two, you can prepare sauces using plain yogurt or low-fat or fat-free sour cream. You can also use dry wine, nuts, seeds, or Parmesan cheese but they should be used sparingly and infrequently, as they are loaded with calories.

Avoid commercial toppings, which generally contain fats, cream, whipped cream, sugar, flour, and other starches, not to mention various chemical substances. When dining out, request that sauces and dressings be served on the side, so that you can control the amounts—and use it sparingly! You can ask what the sauce contains and then decide whether to eat it, use a smaller amount, order a different sauce, or forgo it altogether. Remember that the addition of a fatty sauce can easily double or triple the caloric value of the dish.

20. Take a Multivitamin, Plus Calcium

You should take one balanced multivitamin pill a day, plus a calcium supplement of 600 milligrams to 1,000 milligrams combined with vitamin D. I recommend this as an extra precaution since many foods, including vegetables and fruits, are heavily processed and engineered so that some of the precious vitamins and minerals are lost. Both supplements should be taken with food, while the calcium is better taken with the evening meal. If you have medical problems, you should consult your physician or registered dietitian about vitamin consumption.

STAGE ONE

Stage One of *The Bread for Life Diet* is designed to maximize your weight loss while minimizing your hunger, so it consists mainly of eating bread. That means you should think sandwiches. Tasty, interesting, diverse sandwiches. Lots of them. All throughout the day.

Add some extra taste to your sandwiches by using one of the suggested spreads on pages 83 and 84, then pile on the vegetables, or have a side salad or vegetable soup.

Most people love the idea of eating sandwiches—and lots of them, too—on a diet. Plus, it is so easy to make them because there is no fuss. They also leave you feeling satisfied without feeling heavy, and they will put you in a good mood.

Stage One should be maintained for 1 to 2 weeks only, no more. You can always come back to it later when you need to speed up your weight loss. For some people this stage can get boring no matter how tasty the sandwiches are, but most people love this stage. The latter are usually the people who take advantage of the variety of choices on the diet. I encourage you to make your own choices and experience the variety of offerings. Only when you have freedom to choose your food can you maintain the diet for a lifetime.

This stage was designed for ease and convenience:

+ You can choose from many foods that you like.

+ You don't have to count calories.

+ The rules are easy to follow.

+ Permitted foods are readily available and accessible.

+ You can eat at home, at work, in a restaurant, at parties.

+ You should never be hungry.

+ You'll have energy and be in a good mood.

+ You eat all day long.

+ You can even eat before bedtime.

What You Can Eat

+ Bread—and lots of it! Eight to 12 slices of light bread a day for a woman, and 12 to 16 slices for a man. You can substitute every 2 slices of light bread with 1 slice of ordinary bread or 1 light roll.

+ A thin layer of any spread that is not sweet for each slice of bread.

+ Unlimited amounts of vegetables, with the exception of potatoes, sweet potatoes, and corn.

+ 1 serving of fruit a day, preferably with a low glycemic index. You can substitute the fruit with a dietetic dairy pudding or unsugared, low-fat yogurt.

+ Three to four eggs a week prepared any way you like, with or without bread in the same meal.

- Two to three tablespoons (not teaspoons) of olive or canola oil a day.

- Seven to eight 8-ounce glasses of nonsugared, nonalcoholic fluids a day for women, and eight to nine glasses daily for men.

- Lean meat or fish in unlimited (but reasonable) quantities three times a week with vegetables but no bread or other carbohydrates *in the same meal.* On these three days, reduce your bread quota by 2 to 4 slices of light bread, but do not eat less than 6 slices total for women and 10 slices total for men.

- Take one multivitamin and one calcium plus vitamin D supplement a day.

DINING OUT

Eating in a restaurant is easy even during Stage One. This is when you should take advantage of your meat meal. For example, you can order the following:

- Filet mignon

- Tossed mixed salad with low-fat dressing or olive oil and vinegar on the side

- Asparagus

OR

- Vegetable soup

- Grilled salmon with broccoli

- Tomato, red onion, pepper, and cucumber salad

A SAMPLE DAY IN STAGE ONE

The actual time of day of each meal is not what's important, but eating every 3 to 4 hours *is* important. Arrange your eating schedule according to your lifestyle. The hours given here are only for reference.

Meal 1: 8:00–10:00 A.M.

✦ A sandwich made with 2 slices of toasted light bread with a thin layer of low-fat cottage cheese and slices of tomatoes and peppers

✦ Coffee with artificial sweetener and a little bit of milk (up to 2% fat)

Meal 2: 11:00 A.M.–1:00 P.M.

✦ A sandwich made with 2 slices of light bread, 1 or 2 slices of turkey, mustard, lettuce, and tomatoes

Meal 3: 2:00–4:00 P.M.

✦ Bowl of vegetable soup

✦ 2 slices of light bread

Meal 4: 5:00–7:00 P.M.

✦ A sandwich made with 2 slices of light bread and 1 or 2 slices of low-fat Swiss cheese

✦ A dish of raw or steamed vegetables

Meal 5: 8:00–10:00 P.M.

+ Sandwich made with 2 slices of light bread with a scrambled egg and piled high with vegetables

Meal 6: 11:00 P.M. or later

+ 1 cup of artificially sweetened low-fat yogurt

OR

+ 1 serving of fruit or 1 slice of light bread with a thin spread of choice

Make Sure to:

+ Eat your full allotment of bread.

+ Eat a fish, poultry, and meat meal three times a week with vegetables, but no bread or other starches in the same meal. Reduce your daily light bread quota by two slices.

+ Get 2 to 3 tablespoons of canola or olive oil a day.

+ Eat no more than a single serving of fruit once a day.

+ Drink enough liquids.

+ Take your daily multivitamin and calcium supplements.

Other Meal Ideas

+ 2 slices of light bread with a thin layer of fat-free cream cheese, a piece of smoked salmon, lettuce, and tomatoes

+ A 1-egg omelet with mushrooms and onions, cucumber and tomato salad, and a slice of whole-grain bread

+ 1 cup low-fat plain yogurt with pieces of cucumber and spices

STAGE TWO

Stage Two is based on the principles of Stage One, but is expanded and enriched with many other foods. Variety and correct food selection are the keys to continuing *The Bread for Life Diet* successfully. You can even indulge in a few "forbidden" foods occasionally without feeling guilty.

Some people find it easier to implement Stage One, with its clear rules and simplicity, but few can (and nobody needs to) stick with such a limited selection of foods for more than 2 weeks at a time. The rules of Stage Two provide more freedom of choice, but the choice is not unlimited, and self-discipline and commitment are required. The variety and range of possibilities available to you in Stage Two enable you to maintain the diet for an unlimited time period and adopt it as a way of life.

What You Can Eat

✦ **Bread**—The same amount of bread as in Stage One—8 to 12 slices of light bread for women, 12 to 16 for men—but you can substitute some or all of the bread with other complex carbohydrates that are similar to bread in terms of their composition and quantity. Feel free to substitute other bread choices but follow the "substitution" guide on page 81.

You can substitute two slices of *light* bread with:

✦ **Legumes** (1 cup cooked)—This includes lentils, white or black beans, peas, broad beans, whole chick-peas, and so forth. Legumes have many merits:

  ✦ They contain a combination of starch and protein.

  ✦ Their glycemic index is fairly low.

✦ They are rich in dietary fiber.

✦ They are rich in vitamins and minerals.

Legumes can be used to prepare varied and tasty, hot or cold dishes, but they do have one disadvantage—they are liable to cause gas. Sometimes leaving the legumes on a damp towel or in cold water overnight before cooking them can help.

✦ **Rice** (⅔ to 1 cup cooked)—Anything but white rice. This includes basmati rice, wild rice, and whole-grain rice. They have a lower glycemic index than round-shaped types of white rice. You can eat rice with legumes; in soup; as a stuffing (together with vegetables) for bell peppers, zucchini, grape leaves, or tomatoes; in a Chinese- or Thai-style dish; or in sushi. Avoid rice noodles, found in Chinese cuisine, because of their high glycemic index.

✦ **Pasta** (1 cup cooked)—Pasta made from durum wheat or whole wheat is preferable to white pasta because of its lower glycemic index. When you eat pasta, it is important to choose the right sauce, that is, one without cream, butter, or cheese. Fatty sauces can double or triple the caloric value of a meal. Therefore, the sauces I recommend are tomato sauce, soy sauce, and olive oil, all with or without herbs.

You should eat pasta as a main dish, not a side dish, and you can add all the vegetables you want.

✦ **Grains** (⅔ to 1 cup cooked)—These include pearl barley, millet, buckwheat, oats, or any type of whole grain that can be found at the market. By the way, shopping for grains can be a lot of fun. You can find a variety of grains in all different colors, and they are very tasty as a meal. The glycemic index of most whole grains (not crushed) is quite low. They contain dietary fiber, vitamins, and minerals, and you can use them to prepare other foods such as soups and breakfast cereals.

✦ **Sweet potato** (1 medium-sized)—Sweet potatoes can be boiled, oven-baked, or cooked in the microwave. You can sauté them in a small amount of olive or canola oil. Sweet potatoes contain fiber and the vitamin beta-carotene, and their glycemic index is not high.

✦ **Potato** (1 medium-sized)—You can have potatoes only occasionally due to their high glycemic index. Eat them boiled oven-baked or cooked. Mashed potatoes (especially with butter/margarine) and French fries (deep-fried in oil) are not recommended. In order to improve the vitamin C content and the glycemic index, eat potatoes with the peel on (wash thoroughly). You can sauté potatoes in a very small amount of olive or canola oil.

✦ **Corn** (1 ear, ⅔ cup kernels, or 2 cups popped)—The glycemic index of corn is fairly high, which puts it on the limited-items list. If you love popcorn, eat the air-popped variety, not the kind that uses much oil. Do not butter the popcorn or use the ready-made products that are buttered.

✦ **Breakfast cereals** (4–5 tablespoons)—Cereal can be a substitute for bread but only occasionally because breakfast cereals generally contain sugars, and often contain dried fruit, honey, nuts, or other fattening ingredients. The healthful image of breakfast cereal offers the illusion of being so healthy that you can eat all you like.

Breakfast cereals that can substitute for bread are those that do not contain sugar or other additives but do contain fiber, such as Bran Flakes, All-Bran, or Fiber One. Cornflakes, even without added sugar, have a very high glycemic index, so go easy on how much you eat.

You can have 4 to 5 tablespoons of bran flakes or 2 to 3 tablespoons of cornflakes without sugar (you can use artificial sweetener) as a substitute for two slices of light bread. Be sure to count any milk or yogurt you eat with the breakfast cereal as part of the one-cup daily quota.

✦ **Muesli and granola** (1–2 tablespoons)—You may occasionally have 1 to 2 tablespoons of muesli or granola, but the more rarely the better. There are many types to choose from; try the simplest ones. Since they have a high sugar count, you may have them as a dessert food.

✦ **Crackers, pretzels, rice cakes, and other snacks** (2 or 3 pieces)—Look for whole-wheat crackers and oat crackers, as their substitution value is one to one. Since there is a large variety of these products, it's important to read the nutritional information on the labels, which shows the number of calories that each product contains. This will help you choose carefully and not get carried away. As a rule of thumb, consider every 35 to 45 calories as a substitute for one slice of light bread.

Vegetables—Eat all kinds (except potatoes, sweet potatoes, and corn), without limitation.

Meat, poultry, and fish—Eat lean meat, poultry, seafood, and fish three times a week. If you especially enjoy this type of meal, you may eat it up to five times. You are not limited to an amount, but you should eat reasonable servings. As with Stage One, however, do not have any bread or other carbohydrates in the same meal, only vegetables. Also, on these days, reduce your bread intake to 6 to 8 slices for women and up to 10 for men.

You can eat these protein meals at lunchtime or in the evening, depending on your personal preference and daily schedule. If you are going to a restaurant or to an event, save this type of meal for those times. You can occasionally eat meat, poultry, seafood, or fish twice in the same day. This is not a disaster, just an event that can happen once in a while.

Fruit—There is no problem if you stay with one serving a day. If you are a fruit lover, and your weight loss rate is satisfactory, you can eat two or even three daily fruit servings between meals or as a separate meal, but do note that this may easily slow your weight loss rate or even make you gain weight. Do not eat all your servings in one sitting or as dessert to another meal. If you choose to eat a third serving, it must be as a substitute for one slice of light bread. Choose fruits with a lower glycemic index.

You do not have to eat all the fruit permitted each day. In fact, you do not have to eat fruit at all. It is best to eat it only when you feel a particular need to have it. If you notice that the extra fruits slow your weight loss, return to one a day or forgo them.

There are many people, myself included, who love fruit and find it particularly hard to give up. But on *The Bread for Life Diet*, it is better to give up fruit than skip a meal or not get the required carbohydrates.

Each fruit may be substituted with a dietetic dairy pudding or plain yogurt.

Eggs—You may have one egg, three to four times a week.

Dairy products—You may add some low-fat hard or soft cheese or an extra container of yogurt as a substitute for two slices of light bread. Of course, fat-free products and products with fewer than 1.4 grams of fat per ounce (28 grams) are preferred. If you notice that the extra dairy products slow your weight loss, forgo them.

It is a good idea to eat yogurt a few times a week, if not daily, because it is enriched with calcium. People who are lactose-intolerant can drink a glass of calcium-enriched soy milk instead. The sweet soy puddings that have appeared lately contain a lot of sugar and are not recommended as part of the diet, but tofu (up to 3 to 4 ounces per day) is a great addition, especially if it is calcium-enriched. Remember, if you like your dairy or soy products sweet, make sure you use artificial sweeteners only.

Oil and sauces—As in Stage One, it is important to get 2 to 3 tablespoons a day. Please refer to Pages 95–96 for more details.

Alcohol—Men who enjoy alcoholic beverages are permitted up to 5 drinks a week. Women are permitted up to 3 drinks. A drink is equivalent to:

+ 4 ounces of wine.

+ One 12-ounce bottle of beer (not malt beer, because it contains a lot of sugar).

+ 1 ounce of hard liquor with a noncaloric mixer such as club soda.

Liqueurs are not permitted because they contain added sugar. And keep in mind that alcohol contains a lot of calories. Just because alcohol is permitted does not mean that it is recommended. If you can do without alcohol, it's much preferable.

Desserts—You can have up to 2 ounces of artificially sweetened low-fat ice cream (without a cone) or dairy pudding, but both do contain calories. These can be substituted at any time for a serving of fruit. Sugar-free freezer pops with 8 to 10 calories may be eaten freely. You can also freely enjoy low-calorie Jell-O. You can add some sliced fruit to your Jell-O to make it more delicious.

Treat yourself—Although I recommend not eating protein and carbohydrates together in one meal, you can relax this rule from time to time on Stage Two. If you do want a burger on a bun on occasion, then go for it. Just keep it an occasional treat. If you prefer a meal containing a larger amount of meat, then have it with vegetables only, or have your carbohydrates with vegetables only. If you can be satisfied with a small amount of protein food, you can add 2 to 3 tablespoons of carbohydrates (rice, pasta, beans, barley, and so on). The principle is to make the meal relatively small so you don't raise your insulin too high. Vegetables are free.

If you like to cook, you'll find that *The Bread for Life Diet* offers a great opportunity to prepare special, satisfying gourmet dishes that are suitable for everyone—family, children, and guests. And what could be more pleasant and satisfying than the feeling that you served healthy and tasty food to the people you love? Eating a slightly larger amount on occasion doesn't matter. At worst, you'll lose weight more slowly.

A SAMPLE DAY IN STAGE TWO

Don't think of these meals as breakfast, lunch, and dinner. Think of each of them as a meal unto itself. They can be eaten in any order (e.g., the one listed as third can be eaten as the first), and the same meal can be repeated. Drink seven to nine 8-ounce glasses of water throughout the day and don't skip meals.

If you begin your first meal early in the morning, you may have up to 6 meals a day. If you are hungrier in the early hours, you can eat more frequently (every 2 to 3 hours) and then less frequently in the afternoon (every 4 to 5 hours), or vice-versa. It is up to you. You are the boss and the one who decides when to eat. The important thing is not to skip a meal so you never reach a state of hunger!

The hours are given only as examples:

Meal 1: 7:00–10:00 A.M.

   ✦ 2 slices of toasted light bread with a thin layer of low-fat cottage cheese, avocado, or tahini, and slices of tomato and sweet pepper

✦ Coffee with artificial sweetener and a little bit of milk (up to 2% fat)

OR

✦ ¼ cup bran flakes in ⅔ cup milk (up to 2% fat)

Meal 2: 10:00 A.M.–1:00 P.M.

✦ Salad made of tomatoes, cucumbers, and sweet peppers mixed with a little bit of olive oil and spices

✦ 2 slices of light bread with a slice of turkey and mustard

OR

✦ Tuna salad with lettuce, tomatoes, onions, carrots, and cucumbers

Meal 3: 2:00–5:00 P.M.

✦ One sandwich with avocado and vegetables

✦ Coffee with artificial sweetener and a little bit of milk (up to 2% fat)

OR

✦ A dish from the Bread for Life Recipes, beginning on page 187.

OR

✦ Vegetable soup and two zucchini stuffed with rice and vegetables with stir-fried vegetables

Meal 4: 5:00–8:00 P.M.

+ Chinese stir-fried chicken and vegetables

OR

+ 1 grilled chicken breast

+ Mixed green salad

OR

+ 1 cup low-fat dairy product (e.g., natural yogurt) with radishes and cucumbers

Meal 5: 8:00–11:00 P.M.

+ 1 egg fried in a small amount of olive or canola oil

+ 2 slices of light bread

+ Tomato, red onion, and basil salad

OR

+ 1 cup of cooked pasta with tomato sauce

+ Cabbage salad mixed with a little bit of olive oil and spices

OR

+ 1 serving fruit

OR

+ 1–2 slices of light bread with a thin spread of choice

Meal 6: 11:00 P.M. or later

✦ 1 serving of fruit

OR

✦ 1–2 slices of light bread with a thin spread of choice

THE BREAD FOR LIFE DIET A unique principle of *The Bread for Life Diet* is that you do not reduce the amount of food as you go along. On the contrary, you vary the foods you eat and increase the amounts. If you start eating too much and stop losing weight, or gain weight, you can always switch back to the Stage One menu to get you back on track again and lose weight. As a general rule, it's a good idea to go back to Stage One occasionally in order to maintain or speed up weight loss.

8

Genetics & the Environment

In our affluent world, too much food and too little physical activity are the chief contributing factors to the growing obesity epidemic worldwide and in America in particular. The biological nature of weight gain, however, makes this problem a bit more complex. As anyone with a weight problem probably has jealously noticed, some people can consume a lot of food and remain thin, while others consume very little and still gain weight.

So what's the story? What actually makes us put on pounds? Strange as it may seem, it is more natural for our body to store fat than to actually use it up, which is one reason it is so hard to lose weight. When we go on a diet, we eventually act against this inherent body mechanism.

Excess weight, or more precisely, the body's ability to store fat, developed in ancient times as a survival mechanism when our ancestors had to undergo long periods of food deprivation (famine) alternating with short periods of abundance (feast). In search of food, they used up a lot of energy hunting their prey or traveling long distances to find more fertile soils. Those who were blessed with the ability to store fat during times of abundance used those stores to provide their bodies with energy and sustenance when food became scarce. Thus, they won the struggle for survival.

THE REAL DEAL

There are several causes for weight gain, among them:

+ Heredity, over which we have no control (including genetic diseases leading to extreme obesity).

+ Environment, which we have the power to influence to some degree.

+ Behavior, which we can modify even though sometimes change seems impossible.

+ Metabolic problems, which are beyond the scope of this book, including diseases such as hypothyroidism, excess cortisone production, or an imbalance of sex hormones (for example, polycystic ovary syndrome).

+ Medicines, such as antidepressants and steroids.

Women, whose biological function was to propagate and nurture children for the next generation, evolved their ability to store fat even further than men. In prehistoric society, a woman might become pregnant almost every 9 months, so from an early age, constant pregnancy and nursing made it more difficult for her to do much foraging. If she had no one who could dependably supply her with food (the family structure developed at a relatively late era), this ability to store fat became absolutely necessary to her survival. Without it, she would starve to death. Her genetic legacy, which included evolutionary adaptations of the female hormonal system that supported fat storage, has been passed down through the generations. That's why women "excel" in their increased ability to store fat today.

HEREDITY IS NOT THE FINAL WORD

The ability to store fat has been imprinted in our genetic code as a means of survival and, thanks to these genes, you are reading this book and cursing heredity. Yes, there is such a thing as obesity genes and people who have them gain weight easily and find it very hard to lose, even when following their diet "by the book" and exercising regularly. Nevertheless, these people can choose whether to become helpless victims of heredity and give up their efforts, or work harder and achieve real results.

Our genetic code determines our individual characteristics, but not all of them express themselves during a person's lifetime. Certain environmental factors determine which characteristics are expressed and which are not. These include the quality and amount of food we eat; the burden of physical work we perform; our living and sanitary conditions; the quality of health services available to us; work, rest, and stress conditions; our level of education; and so on.

For example, the average height among people in developed countries has increased over the years. Why? Because the living conditions of children have improved, and they could reach their full growth potential. Under

GENES PLAY A BIG ROLE

When researchers examined weight gain among identical twins who had been separated during childhood and grew up in different foster families, they discovered an interesting pattern. Even though they lived in different environments, twins often tended to have a similar pattern of gaining or not gaining weight over the years.

The role heredity plays in obesity also shows itself among children of overweight or thin parents. If one parent is overweight, the probability of his or her child being overweight is approximately 40 percent. If both parents are overweight, it increases to approximately 80 percent; and in families where both parents are thin, the probability of a child being overweight drops to less than 20 percent.

poor environmental conditions (a lack of food, shelter, or sanitation), people can't reach their genetic potential for height, so they remain shorter.

Excess weight works in the same way. A genetic tendency to gain weight exists, but it can be fully expressed only under suitable environmental conditions, such as an abundance of available food and a sharp drop in physical activity. According to recently published research, only 8 percent of the immigrants who had lived in the United States for less than a year were obese, but that number jumped to 19 percent among those who had been living in the United States for at least 15 years.

The Pima Indians in the Southwest are another example. Those in the tribe who live in Mexico, where they consume a traditional diet (less animal fat, more complex carbohydrates) and are more physically active, have a much lower prevalence of obesity and type 2 diabetes than do those living in Arizona. People of the Arizona branch of the tribe consume an "Americanized" diet (high in fat and low in complex carbohydrates and fiber) and are much less physically active. Of the 7,000 Pima Indians living today in Arizona, more than 75 percent are obese and 45 percent have type 2 diabetes.

It seems that all of America may reach these figures in the not too distant future if steps are not taken to stop the trend. According to the most recent United States census figures, 34 percent (68.3 million) of U.S. adults age 20 and above are overweight (BMI of 25 to 30) and 30.5 percent (61.3 million) are obese (a BMI of above 30).

Men are heavier (67.2 percent) than women (61.9 percent) but more women are considered obese (33.4 percent) than men (27.6 percent). Also, 15.3 percent of children and 15.5 percent of adolescents are overweight or obese. Another 15 percent are considered at risk for being overweight.

This is a real epidemic! So, what's going on? It is popular to blame heredity, but the genetics have always been there. So why now, of all times, are entire populations getting fatter?

One reason is our "good fortune" for having an unprecedented, huge variety of fattening and easily accessible foods. Another is that modern technology has made it possible for us to do many daily routines with much less physical effort. We "hunt" for food at one-stop markets. We get to the hunting grounds by car where we fight for the space closest to the door. Sometimes we forage without even leaving the house, by telephone or over the Internet.

These same laid-back conditions can trigger other destructive genetic tendencies as well. Type 2 diabetes is a good example. By 1991, 5 percent of Americans over age 20 had diagnosed diabetes. By 2002, the figure was nearly 9 percent—almost double. Yet, this type of diabetes is preventable, no matter what your genes. Excess weight is the major cause; maintaining healthy weight, healthy food intake, and regular physical activity is the solution.

CONTROLLING YOUR ENVIRONMENT

No one has to give in to their genes. We all have the ability to influence or even shift our genetic predisposition, and the result can be profound. For example, if we cultivate the intellect of a not particularly brilliant child, he or she might grow up to be a professor; without suitable cultivation, even the most brilliant child can end up a homeless drug addict.

The rate of childhood obesity in America is alarming. According to government statistics, obesity among preschoolers is 10 percent! We're talking about children 2 to 5 years old, almost totally dependent upon their parents for making their food choices. Is it just heredity? Or could it be junk food, too much television and computer games, and too little active recreation outside? Or is it that family meals have become so rare that parents don't get to see what their children eat?

It is easy to recognize the impact environmental factors, such as these habits, are having on children. We cannot control a child's heredity, so when parents who are overweight bring their overweight offspring to me for consultation, I get them to focus on changing the child's environment, the family's lifestyle, and the parents' eating and food-purchasing behavior. In cases like this, outlining a diet for the child is not enough. Without a change in the eating patterns of the entire family, chances of success are slim. Today's children have to cope with too many outside influences, so good food habits have to begin at home.

Here's an example. A mother came to me with her overweight 10-year-old son who was ashamed of his body because other children mocked him and called him insulting names. During our conversation, I found out that his mother kept a locked drawer filled with candy, and every family member, except the boy, was permitted access to the drawer. It was very difficult to convince the mother that her strategy was less than effective, as it only left her son feeling isolated and deprived, and made him long for candy even more. After all, he was just as much a member of the family as anyone else in their home and he should be permitted to eat whatever everyone else ate.

In cases like this one, I suggest a method that is more effective than prohibitions and locks: Set uniform rules that apply equally to everyone in the family. It can be one candy a day or candy only on weekends. Allow no one any candy over and above that.

GOOD INTENTIONS?

Sometimes I suggest to parents that they ban candy and cake from the home, according to the idea that "Giving a thousand kisses is better than giving a thousand cookies." If we learn to express love by means other than offering food, such as giving gifts, watching television together, talking with each other, and spending quality time together, we can create a warm and wonderful home environment without putting our children's and our own weight and health at risk.

A father came to see me for help with his overweight 10-year-old daughter. She was doing well on the eating routine that I gave her and was happy with her weight loss. And the father? He began to secretly offer her biscuits out of pity for her "misery!" And he did it as an act of love! No wonder so many children find it difficult to control their weight.

There is little harm in buying a chocolate bar once in a while when away from home or ordering a dessert in the restaurant. These occasions are relatively few compared to having sweets in the house. And it teaches your children that sweets are something special to be enjoyed on special occasions.

Weight loss begins at home. If you can't deal with your own weight, you can't expect to be successful at helping a child deal with a weight problem.

The Bread for Life Diet is a healthy lifestyle plan that works for the entire family. The best way to help an overweight child is to teach by example.

This way, children learn to eat what the family eats, rather than a "special diet" that is perceived by the child as punishment. *The Bread for Life Diet* will instill healthy nutritional behavior.

THE BREAD FOR LIFE DIET cannot change your genes, but it can help you change your environment. It will guide you in choosing the right foods for you and for your family.

9

Changing Behaviors: The Six Insights

We eat for many reasons. Most have nothing to do with being hungry or satisfying physiological needs. In fact, people who eat only when they're hungry generally fall into four groups: babies, toddlers under the age of about 3, adolescent boys, and thin men. Most of us eat for reasons other than just sustenance.

We eat to reward ourselves on a particularly good day. We eat to console ourselves on a particularly bad day. We eat for instant gratification when we feel bad, sad, or depressed; after an unpleasant conversation with the boss, spouse, or a friend; for a boost when we feel tired; and for consolation when things don't go as expected. In fact, any difficulty in daily routine can call for solace in the form of food.

Many people prefer it to other means of emotional escape, such as smoking, alcohol, medication, drugs, or sex. Food is the ultimate pacifier.

We may find some comfort in eating that extra serving or two, but does it really make us feel better in the long run? Of course not. More often than not, it makes us feel guilty. So what do we do? Eat more! Food becomes both crime and punishment, as we discover when we look in the mirror or step on the scale.

If this behavior typifies you, my intention is not to make you feel bad. It is common among people who have a weight issue. But it is a destructive behavioral pattern that needs to be broken. And it can be broken. When I meet with patients to discuss their dieting issues, I don't just give them a list of foods to eat and send them off. I discuss destructive eating problems and coach them in what I call the "Six Insights."

THE FIRST INSIGHT

Nothing in life is black and white, including dieting!

There is no point in putting 100 percent of your effort into a diet then giving up completely if you don't have 100 percent success. Between black and white there are colors and shades, and you need to find your niche among them. Nothing in life is black and white, including dieting!

The "all or nothing" principle does not work to your advantage. It works to your disadvantage, and to tell you the truth, it will often trick you into failure. If you eat something that is not in the diet, just remember that it is not the ruination of your diet. There is no reason to punish yourself. After all, you are not a computer or robot or some kind of machine; you are allowed and expected to slip up occasionally. All you did was eat something that was not included in the diet, which is expected to happen, and that's perfectly all right!

Accept it as part of the process, continue your efforts at weight loss, and give up any feelings of guilt you may have. If such feelings arise, and they will arise, tell yourself that you will not break your diet out of guilt because there is nothing to be guilty about. Just continue with your diet as if nothing happened. This self-talk can be very effective. It can support you in maintaining weight loss and a stable weight in the long term.

Missions are for the army and the FBI, not for individuals. Treat yourself gently, allow for gradual progress, and don't punish or rebuke yourself for being less than perfect. Moreover, I often ask those of my patients who are struck with guilt to deliberately have a piece of cake or some ice cream once in a while. It helps get them in the mindset that it is not breaking their diet. This practice makes people feel great and it helps them enjoy the diet and allows them to pick up where they left off after a "slip-up." Do not be afraid to step out of the diet once in a while. It makes it possible to go on with the eating program. The worst that can happen is that your weight loss will be slower. So what? There's no hurry.

THE SECOND INSIGHT

Accept yourself and come to terms with who you really are.

This does not mean patting yourself on the back for being overweight. Rather, if you internalize the fact that you have a genetic tendency toward overweight or obesity, you'll accept the reality that you must invest a greater effort to lose weight than does someone upon whom God did not bestow these genes.

After all, denial does not make the issue go away. You are who you are, whether you accept it or not. Whether you accept being overweight or deny it, your genes won't change. If you don't accept this fact, you will always be searching for someone or something to blame. "There must be something wrong with the diet, or the dietitian, or the therapist, or life, or the world."

With this kind of attitude, you'll only try to follow more and more diets in search of the perfect solution, but you will never succeed. Your goal should be to get down to a healthy weight, not to be rail thin like a model. If you accept the fact that, "I have a weight problem and must be careful about what I eat" you can quickly progress to the point of, "I am prepared to do what is necessary to change the situation, even if it is harder for me than for other people." You can't solve a problem if you don't admit there is one.

The motto that we should adopt for making changes in general, and a diet change in particular, is "I am the way I am, and I am responsible for what I am going to be." It is the starting point for positive change.

You can perceive the tendency to be overweight as a tragedy and become a victim of it. Alternatively, you can accept is as a part of reality, as the way things are, and not expect your body to behave other than the way it does. Given that, you can start doing what it takes to lose weight, without expecting it to be as easy or as hard as it might be for others. Accepting the situation is not an exemption from any effort, but an incentive for making the effort, and succeeding!

THE THIRD INSIGHT

The flavor of a single square of chocolate is identical to the flavor of the whole bar.

Many of my patients use this simple but crafty insight as their everyday mantra. And it works! It is part of how to win at losing and maintaining weight. People with this insight can go to a wedding or any event that offers an abundance of food and limit themselves to a single taste of this or even steal a teaspoon of that from their partner and say: "It tastes the same as the whole piece."

THE FOURTH INSIGHT

There are many obstacles on the road to successful weight loss, but each and every one can be identified and overcome.

Simply deciding to go on a diet or begining one is no guarantee of ultimate success, because reality poses endless traps and mines that will divert your success. Only if you know how to identify these obstacles and learn how to deal with them will you be able to overcome them.

Here are a few common examples with suggestions on how to overcome some of the obstacles. Obviously, choose a method that best suits you.

Eating without paying attention to what you're eating. We often eat while paying no attention to what and how much food we're actually consuming. Instead, we engage in various other activities that distract us from paying attention to our meal, such as talking on the telephone, studying, reading a book or a newspaper, working at the computer, or watching television.

My solution is two-fold: First, devote a specific time and place to eating, during which you can give it your exclusive attention. If you find yourself eating while you're engaged in another activity, either stop eating or abandon the other activity. Second, write down the name and amount of every bit of food that goes into your mouth immediately upon eating it. If you wait until later, you will forget—trust me. All of this bookkeeping is particularly helpful in becoming aware of the little things you eat, like peanuts, sunflower seeds, potato chips, or tiny cookies, which don't seem to count but are actually big in terms of calories.

Many people think that keeping a food diary is a boring, burdensome, and irritating task. Perhaps it is, but you can use it to your advantage. Assuming you don't want to cheat, you can avoid tedious writing by not eating that one extra thing. Besides, writing everything down gives you an extra opportunity to consider whether you really want to eat a particular food or not. And, at the end of the day, you'll have a detailed picture of everything you ate.

You may be surprised at what you learn. You'll most likely find that you've been eating foods that really aren't necessary for your health, survival, or even pleasure. You can avoid those foods the following day. But even without conscious effort, you'll find yourself almost automatically reducing the amount of food you eat, which will in turn contribute to your weight loss. I employ this technique occasionally myself when I feel that I am neglecting my diet. Some of my patients use this technique to remind themselves of the successful food choices they made on previous days.

Excessive eating at special events. Do you ever find yourself "saving" calories for a whole day, knowing that in the evening there will be lots of tasty, free food at a party, banquet, or reception you'll be attending? Not a good idea. You'll end up eating way too much.

The solution: If you do not want to be hungry in the evening, you must eat normally during the day. Moreover, it is a good idea to have something tasty and filling to eat just before you leave for the event. If you don't arrive hungry, you have much more control over what you eat. Making food choices that work for your weight and health will be far easier, and you can still enjoy sample tasting the wonderful fare that's offered.

Do you sometimes find yourself loading up your plate with so much food that you can hardly finish it all? Remember the mantra of the Third Insight: The flavor of a single square of chocolate is identical to the flavor of the whole bar. Your eyes really can be bigger than your stomach.

One successful tactic is to begin your meal by drinking a glass of water or a diet drink. Then select a salad or vegetable soup as a first course. This way you'll reduce your hunger before the other courses arrive. Keep in mind that you are not a child anymore. You won't be punished for not finishing everything on your plate.

Excessive eating in the evening and at night. If you find yourself eating after dinner or at night, the reason could be fatigue, real hunger, or a drop in your serotonin level.

One solution for getting through what I call "the dangerous hours" is to have on hand lots of cut-up vegetables, low-calorie Jell-O, and less-fattening snacks such as rice cakes, crisp crackers, or popcorn with no oil or butter. Or, you can opt for a larger meal in the evening instead of the afternoon. It is also a good idea to go for a walk in the evening or engage in other sports activities, which will refresh and energize you, and make those hunger pangs disappear.

This should not be a big problem on *The Bread for Life Diet* because you spread the meals throughout your waking hours, including late hours and before going to sleep

Strong cravings for something sweet after lunch. Find yourself craving desserts after your midday meal? You may have a conditioned reflex, a need to feel pampered, a need to vent, or a physiological response to a rise in insulin, or a drop in serotonin level. This is common after eating meat because protein can make serotonin go down and a big meal can make insulin go up.

One solution to satisfy these cravings is to have on hand a nonfattening dessert, such as low-calorie Jell-O, a slice of melon, or a serving of some other fruit. Try to postpone eating it for at least an hour after the meal. You can also try eating smaller meals, as large meals make you more prone to want something sweet.

Tasting while you're cooking. My question is, "Is this the first time you have cooked this dish?" Probably not. There is no need to taste dishes you've prepared many times before. You already know what they taste like, so give up this excuse and profit by losing weight. This does not mean that tasting is forbidden. If you must check to make sure a dish is turning out the way it's supposed to, then all you really need is a tiny taste.

Not being able to say "no" to an offer of food. "The hostess offered me a piece of cake she made, and I felt uncomfortable saying no, so I ate it." I hear it all the time. But when I reply, "Had you been offered a fried snake, would you have eaten it because you felt uncomfortable saying no?"

Politeness is the perfect excuse to rationalize giving in to the strong desire to eat. After the initial sense of pleasure has worn off, however, what generally remains is a feeling of guilt and disappointment, which often leads to abandoning the diet altogether. It is better to stop yourself before sinking your teeth into that cake.

Instead of creating an excuse in favor of indulging yourself, you can usually get off the hook by saying you have high blood pressure or high cholesterol. Simply saying you are on a diet may not help, as you might encounter responses such as, "No dieting allowed in my house!" But if you stay firm, most people will understand.

There are, however, those who particularly love to press food on people who are on a diet. When this happens, make up a counter-excuse such as, "I'm really stuffed, there was so much delicious food" or some other comment that can not be debated. A convincing answer eventually reduces the pressure. Of course, you might just want to eat the cake without making any excuses. In this case, spare yourself the guilt and the excuse and just enjoy the cake. And after the last bite, go back on your diet.

Buying and bringing home food you can not resist. There are three typical mistakes: The first is buying the food, the second is putting the first piece in your mouth, and the third is continuing to eat, absent-mindedly, until the package is empty. There are three solutions: The first is not to buy it at all, even if the (declared) reason for buying it is for the children or because you are having guests. The second is not to start eating it, not even to taste it. The third is either stop at one; or put a serving on a plate, put the rest back where it belongs, and eat it slowly so you will savor it with your fullest attention.

THE FIFTH INSIGHT

You can be on a diet and still enjoy life.

Many people associate the concept of a diet with a lot of prohibitions, as if they were in prison. That's why most weight-loss diets do not work. Depriving yourself of food only leads to an outburst of hunger, which you feel both physically and emotionally. No wonder you pounce on chocolate bars as if your life depended on them after coming off a rigorous diet.

By the way, this holds true not only for humans. In laboratory tests, animals that had been deprived of food reacted with signs of excessive pleasure the moment they were permitted to eat, and they consumed more food that they normally would.

The solution: Do not skip meals. Do not allow yourself to get hungry. Eat *before* you are hungry. Occasionally *do* eat something that is not recommended. *The Bread for Life Diet* is an opportunity to enjoy your diet, and to feel satisfied physically, mentally, and emotionally. People who have gone on my diet tell me that they stop having cravings for sweets and the like because they are not hungry in the first place. And when they do want something, they are content with having just a taste. You can eat any food, as long as you do not overdo the amounts and frequencies. Thus, *The Bread for Life Diet* becomes a way of life you can easily and pleasurably follow, indeed for life.

THE SIXTH INSIGHT

Excuses and self-justification keep you overweight!

Do any of the following sound like you?

"I asked her not to eat cookies in front of me, and she promised she wouldn't, but she did anyway, so I couldn't help myself."

"He insulted me so deeply! So I ate to console myself, just a little. Wouldn't you? Don't I deserve something good in life?"

"She gets so offended if I don't eat what she makes. She is so proud of her cooking! I can't say no!"

"I eat in restaurants with clients all the time and I have to order all the courses so they can feel free to do so. It would be impolite not to!"

"I just took one peanut, and then I found myself with an empty bag! I don't even know how it happened!"

"I bought the cake for the guests, and they only ate half of it. We don't throw food away."

The more excuses you have and the more you justify your actions, the more they become a natural way of life, and the more likely you'll remain overweight.

A PLAN OF ACTION

If you are reading this book, it means you are interested in losing weight. Hopefully, you are ready to make the commitment to change the way you eat. A real diet has a beginning but there is no end. It means changing your eating style but it does not mean—actually must not mean—you should feel hungry and be miserable. With that in mind, consider the following. Don't get started until you can take these steps with both feet planted firmly in your goal.

Action Step No. 1: You Make the Decision

When a patient comes to me and says, "My wife told me I need to lose weight," I know that there's little point in helping him because he does not have the commitment to make it happen. He does not yet have a personal commitment to himself.

A real decision is not lip service. People procrastinate about doing a lot of things, but putting off a diet is one of the most common. How often have you said, "I'll start a diet tomorrow"?

The process of deliberating over whether to begin a diet or delay it is in a way similar to what happens when we are faced with a sinkful of dirty dishes. We invest a lot of time and energy thinking and pondering whether to tackle the dishes now or to wash them the next day, and this wastes more energy than if we just started washing them.

The decision to go on *The Bread for Life Diet* should not be difficult because it does not feel like a diet. There is no deprivation.

One of my patients said to me: "I'm 40 and I've always been thin until a couple of years ago. It's the first time I'm on any kind of diet, and I was quite concerned that being on a diet would be very unpleasant and demanding. However, when I started *The Bread for Life Diet*, I saw it's not bad at all! It's not even a matter of eating that much less, only choosing the right foods and spreading the meals out so that you're never hungry." He lost some 30 pounds in two months.

Deciding means making a commitment to yourself, to your health, and to your shape. I have often heard people who visit me for the first time say, "It's so hard for me to diet, because I'm weak and have no willpower."

In reply, I tell them that dieting has little to do with lack of willpower. I tell them that, in fact, they have a great deal of willpower. They raise children. They get up every morning to go to work. Some are responsible for tens or hundreds of people. Some make decisions that determine the fate of companies or even of countries. Some work hard days and nights, and others appear on stage every night. Some, especially women, successfully coordinate home and work. Are these the characteristics of a weak character, a shortage of willpower, or a lack of perseverance? Of course not.

People too often associate a diet with suffering, limitations, and missing out on the fun others are having. *The Bread for Life Diet* makes dieting easy, takes the suffering out of dieting, makes it possible to eat with family and friends, to dine out, and to enjoy eating while on vacation. This diet is tailored so you can enjoy living.

Action Step No. 2: Set Realistic Goals

This means taking things slowly and surely. Inflated and difficult goals only lead to frustration and disappointment—the greatest enemies to any weight loss incentive. Setting short-term goals is an effective way to go because you achieve results often. It is a great morale booster. Be happy and encouraged by every achievement, no matter how small it may seem to you, since encouragement and achievement are essential conditions for success.

Dieting is not a game of hero, especially not a suffering hero or a martyr. The weight-loss process inherently is not as fast as we would like it to be. Do not expect fast results. It is better to lose a pound at a time than some of the alternatives: losing none, gaining back, or even losing 2 pounds quickly and gaining 1 or 2 back, quickly or slowly.

Look at your weight reduction from this perspective: Even if you lose "only" a pound a month, you can close a year 12 pounds lighter. Not bad! Besides, there are advantages to losing weight slowly: It's healthier, less muscle tissue is broken down, and your facial features won't sag.

Consider two people who have just weighed themselves after 2 weeks on a diet. Each lost 1 pound. The first says: "That's it?! I tried so hard!" The second says: "I lost a pound! How wonderful!" I don't need to tell you who is more likely to lose more weight.

Don't set goals that represent merely the number of pounds that you want to lose. Instead, set your sights on changing the habits that will enable you to achieve and maintain the weight loss you desire. For example:

+ If you are the type of person who must have three cookies with your afternoon coffee break, your goal is to change this conditioned reflex. The solution is to eat a slice of bread spread with a thin layer of sugar-free jam (fewer calories and more filling).

+ If you eat lunch every day at a restaurant where the hamburgers are superb and you are unhappy eating a salad while everyone is eating burgers, your goal is to find another restaurant where the salads are better than the burgers, or that does not serve burgers at all. If your friends support you, they will go along with you.

+ If you feel that you must eat chocolate after a meat meal, it's probably because that is what you are used to. Your goal is to replace the chocolate with a serving of fruit and to postpone eating the fruit for 1 hour after your meal.

+ If you "attack" your meal, your goal is to start every meal with a green salad. Another goal is to slow the speed at which you usually eat. You can measure how long it takes to eat a meal, and start eating more slowly, chewing each bite more thoroughly, until it takes you twice as long to finish the same amount of food.

+ If you hate cutting up vegetables, and therefore don't eat them at all, your goal is to buy cut-up vegetables or to eat them whole. Weight loss is worth the extra cost.

- If you eat nonstop when you are tired, your goal is to go out for an hour-long walk or to eat one slice of light bread a half-hour before you would usually feel tired, even if you're not hungry.

- If you are constantly tempted by the cookies people bring to the office, and you eat them even though they're not particularly tasty, your goal is to stay away from the break room where the snacks are kept.

Just start small and add one achievement at a time. Just as a baby's first steps cause their parents pride and happiness, you will be proud of yourself for every little step on your new road to success. I know this because not only have I seen this principle work with my patients, but also I have experienced it myself. I remember when I began walking for a half-hour every day. At first I felt bored and annoyed, but gradually I got used to it and, to my surprise, I started to really enjoy my walks. After 3 months, I couldn't imagine not walking!

Another example: I began eating a small sandwich every 3 hours. At first it seemed like a big bother to me, an impossible mission, and I had to keep reminding myself to eat. In time, this habit became a matter of course, without any effort or thinking on my part.

Attaining little goals turns into attaining big goals on the way to losing weight and acquiring new eating habits.

Action Step No. 3: Create Partnerships

Our lives are intertwined with the lives of family, friends, and colleagues. Relationships affect our environment, our eating habits, our self-image, and our behavior. For example, dieters have been known to be on the receiving end of some pretty insulting remarks. A husband who very much wanted his wife to lose weight, for example, used this original way to encourage her: "You look like a cow. It's time to lose weight," and,

"Take a look at yourself, you don't have anything left to wear, everything is too tight on you." There is also the wife who instills motivation in her husband with comments like, "You look like a pig. Do something with yourself." These things really do happen.

Successful dieting is greatly helped by having supportive partners. The concept is simple but can be surprisingly difficult for people to achieve. Rely on your family, friends, colleagues at work, or anyone else who has interest in supporting you. Here are some ways in which your partnerships can help you reach and maintain your weight-loss goals:

✦ Having somebody remind you of your commitment when he or she sees you weakening, reaching for another helping, having "just one" cookie, and so on.

✦ Avoiding situations that are temptations like all-you-can eat buffets.

✦ Joining you for physical activity, such as going for a walk at lunch or bike riding on the weekend.

✦ Avoiding criticism and insulting remarks.

✦ Joining you in the diet.

Here's what to do: Define the situations in which it is hard for you to stay with your diet, and ask a person you trust to support you in this area. Here is a personal example. I like olives, and when they're sitting in front of me, I find it hard to stop eating them until the whole plateful is gone. I asked my daughter to take away the dish with the olives whenever she sees me eating them. Had she done so without being asked, I would have become annoyed and angry. Since she does so at my request, I get less annoyed and ultimately thank her for her concern.

Keep in mind that your health and your diet are solely your responsibility, and nobody else's. Never get angry with your supporters or blame them for your slip-ups. In the end, it is your responsibility to resist temptation and keep yourself on track.

Many of my patients tell me that their entire families not only support them but actually join them in their diet. They discuss which foods to buy and what dishes to prepare. It is very empowering to the person who wants to lose weight. Together with the feeling of partnership and belonging, it often draws families closer. There is a mutual theme for conversation (sometimes the only one), which makes dieting easier to maintain. The truth is that *The Bread for Life Diet* contains so many choices and can be so healthy, pleasant, tasty, and satisfying, that it can work for the entire family for a lifetime.

THE BREAD FOR LIFE DIET takes into account the inevitable difficulties people confront when trying to lose weight and change eating habits, so it offers insights to successfully overcome these obstacles. *The Bread for Life Diet* does not focus on prohibitions; it focuses on permissions. A diet with "stop" signs everywhere is doomed to failure.

10

Energy: It's Still a Balancing Act

The principle of energy balance is simple: It's the difference between how much energy you take in and how much you use up. When these two factors get out of kilter, body weight changes.

It doesn't matter how you try to rationalize weight gain and loss. If you take in more energy than you expend, you gain weight. If you do the opposite, you lose weight. A balance between the energy you expend and the energy you take in will keep you at a steady weight. It is a scientific fact that has not changed since day one.

Your body takes in energy in only one way: as food. Energy is required to keep the body functioning. Muscular activity, growth, replenishing and building of tissues and organs, chemical processes, and regulation of body temperature are among the many functions that depend on energy. Your body burns energy in three main ways: through basal metabolism, through physical activity, and by creating heat as a result of consuming food. And this is where energy balance can differ from person to person.

BASAL METABOLISM

The human body expends energy to maintain itself, even when it is resting. When you are asleep or in a state of deep relaxation, you are less active but your body is using energy to do such things as keeping your heart, kidneys, lungs, and brain functioning as well as maintaining blood flow and body temperature. All these body activities at resting state are called "basal metabolism" and the energy needed to maintain them is called "basal energy expenditure."

To illustrate, let's compare the energy consumption of your body at rest to electricity consumption in your home when you go away for the weekend. Although the house is locked, the refrigerator continues to operate, the light on the television is glowing, and the electric clock is ticking. Will the electric bill disregard this consumption? No, the meter continues to tick, albeit more slowly. Although the electric consumption required to maintain an empty house is low relative to when someone is home (using the dishwasher, cooking, and watching TV), as much as 60 percent of the overall energy your body expends goes to support basal metabolism.

Basal metabolic rate is inherent in a human's genetic hardware. A person with a slower rate of basal metabolism will burn off less energy and that will make him or her gain weight more easily. A person with a faster rate of basal metabolism will burn off more energy, and he or she will have a greater chance of being thin and find it easier to lose weight.

Unfortunately, you don't have much influence when it comes to your basal metabolic rate. The factors that affect it include:

WHY CALORIES AREN'T COUNTED

Food energy is measured in calories. One calorie equals the amount of energy required to raise the temperature of 1 milliliter of water by 1° Celsius. In everyday language, the term calorie (Cal) is used interchangeably with *kilocalorie* (Kcal), which is actually 1,000 calories.

Each gram of consumed proteins or carbohydrates supplies the body with 4 calories, 1 gram of fat supplies 9 calories, and 1 gram of alcohol supplies 7 calories. In other words, the total amount of calories that you consume is equal to the number of grams of each of the three components of food multiplied by the number of calories each component supplies.

Complicated? It can be, especially when you consider that weight gain or loss depends on balancing the calories you take in with the calories you burn. And how effectively calories are burned is different from one person to the next. That's why counting calories is a waste of time.

Since counting calories can't give precise values, there is no calorie counting on *The Bread for Life Diet.* Rather, you eat mainly foods that will burn off energy as a result of the process of consuming food. The diet is designed to burn calories in the most effective ways:

By eating small meals every 3 to 4 hours. By choosing complex carbohydrates that raise your serotonin levels and keep you from being hungry. By sticking with carbohydrates that have a low glycemic index, which prevents your insulin level from rising too much.

Counting calories does not *burn* many, and is not worth the effort.

Muscle mass: The more muscle in your body, the faster your metabolic rate.

Age: At a very young age and during adolescence, especially in teenage boys, the average metabolic rate is fairly rapid and later slows down. After the age of 40, it drops steadily, reinforcing the tendency to gain weight. During old age, muscle mass decreases, and this also affects metabolism.

Gender: Women have a slower metabolic rate than men. This happens, at least in part, because men generally have greater muscle mass. In women over the age of 40, basal metabolism slows down by approximately 3 percent every 5 years; in men it drops about 3 percent every 10 years.

Nutritional manipulations: Fasting and low-calorie crash diets (radical and rapid weight loss) cause the basal metabolic rate to slow down. Have you ever wondered after you've been on various kinds of diets, especially very rigorous ones, why you regain weight so quickly? The answer is that such diets cause your basal metabolic rate to slow down. That's why it is really important to eat when trying to lose weight. Fasting or skipping meals is counterproductive.

Hormones: The thyroid gland is responsible for regulating metabolism and energy burn. A drop in the activity of thyroid hormones will slow down metabolism, which is liable to cause weight gain. A rise in thyroid activity generally does the opposite; it causes an increase in the metabolism rate and weight loss. Some other hormones that affect basal metabolism are the growth hormone (children have a faster metabolism rate), stress hormones such as adrenaline, steroid hormones such as cortisone, and sex hormones such as progesterone.

Smoking: Smokers tend to burn off more calories, but not much more, than nonsmokers. This fact should not be perceived as a recommendation to start smoking, but merely as a partial explanation for the well-known phenomenon of people gaining weight after quitting smoking. Another common reason for this weight gain is that smokers' hands and mouths are busy. When they don't have cigarettes, they use food instead. Nevertheless, *The Bread for Life Diet* is effective for people who have quit smoking.

There are additional factors, such as medication and having a high fever, that may affect metabolic rate, but generally healthy people can speed their metabolism by following *The Bread for Life Diet.*

PHYSICAL ACTIVITY

Some energy is burned off through physical activity—that is, the movement of all or part of your body. Any actions you can think of—talking, arguing, laughing, turning over in bed—are physical activities. Then, of course, there is the physical activity that first comes to mind—exercise.

Unlike basal metabolism, which is determined by your genetic code, physical activity mainly depends on your discipline, awareness, ability, and persistence. It consumes energy not only directly due to burning off calories by performing particular activities, but also indirectly, due to causing an increase in muscle mass. Muscle brings about an increase in basic metabolic rate. This means you will burn calories more efficiently as you continue to lose fat and gain muscle.

Unfortunately, it is our bad luck that a genetic factor is involved here, too. People with a tendency to gain weight expend less energy (relative to their weight) during physical activity than do thin people performing the same activity, so they have to work harder in order to achieve similar results.

It is important to note that our attitude toward the activity we are performing also affects the rate at which we expend energy. For example, a person who spends an hour sitting in a classroom and displays interest and involvement in what is going on burns about 90 calories during that hour. By contrast, a person who sits apathetically and disinterested burns only half of it, just as if he or she were asleep during class. It is no accident that active and enthusiastic people are usually thinner than their opposites. It's more proof that enthusiasm really does count a lot!

GENERATING HEAT

The act of consuming food, which includes the processes of chewing, digestion, breaking down food, absorbing nutrients, and transporting nutrients to the cells of the body, requires energy. It accounts for 10 to 15 percent of our overall basic energy expenditure. The foods that burn off the most energy are proteins and *complex* carbohydrates. Fat in the food has only a very small influence on burning energy. Fat also contains twice the calories of protein and carbohydrates.

If you're interested in counting calories by using food composition tables, you should know that the caloric values stated in these tables are gross values obtained by completely burning foods by fire. The net caloric value of food as obtained by the body is smaller, partly because some energy is used for generating heat as a result of the process of consuming food.

People who choose diets based on fasting, drastically reducing the amount of food they eat, or severely limiting food variety (for example, people who eat only lettuce or only cabbage soup) slow down their basal metabolism, which is counterproductive. And this is in addition to their suffering from hunger, which is common and expected on crash diets. It is important to eat regularly, especially when you're on a diet.

THE NUTRIENT GROUPS

There are 6 main nutrient groups: proteins, carbohydrates, fats, vitamins, minerals, and water. We get our calories from three of them, (proteins, carbohydrates, and fats) as well as from alcohol (which has caloric value but no nutritional value). Vitamins, minerals, and water do not supply energy to the body and do not contain calories. This answers the many people who ask me if vitamins make them put on weight. The answer is no, food does. Eating from each of these groups is essential to your health. Here's why.

Proteins

Proteins are composed of amino acids and are primarily needed for building the body, repairing injuries, and creating enzymes, hormones, and constituents of immune and blood-clotting systems. In short, they keep the body's various cells and tissues functioning.

Proteins come both from animal and vegetable sources, but more are found in animal sources than in vegetable. Protein, however, can be found in almost every food to some extent. The exceptions are sugar and oil.

An excess of proteins turns into fat and increases the fat reservoirs in the body.

Carbohydrates

Carbohydrates are divided into three types: simple carbohydrates (sugars), complex carbohydrates (starches), and dietary fibers. In the digestive system, carbohydrates break down mainly into glucose, a sugar that is essential to every cell in the body. The body does not store carbohydrates, apart from a small amount of glycogen that is found in the liver and muscles. When we fast, glycogen breaks down within approximately 12 hours in order to satisfy the body's immediate energy needs. When we eat too much, excess carbohydrates are turned into fat and go into storage in fat cells until needed.

The list of *simple* carbohydrates (sugars) includes: sucrose (brown and white sugar), fructose (fruit sugar found in a variety of fruits and in corn syrup), glucose (grape sugar), and lactose (milk sugar). Sugars are found in honey, jam, fruit, milk, and in everything to which sugar has been added.

Complex carbohydrates (starches) include all whole grains (wheat, oats, barley, etc.), potatoes, rice, corn, pasta, and legumes. There are two main types of starches—amylose and amylopectin. The proportion between them in food is one of the factors influencing the glycemic index value.

Excess consumption of simple and complex carbohydrates turns them into fat.

Dietary fibers are indigestible components found in vegetables, fruit, grains, and legumes. There are so-called soluble and insoluble fibers. The more fibers (especially soluble) present in the food, the more it influences its glycemic index.

Fats

Fats are made up of fatty acids and constitute a concentrated supply of energy. Some fatty acids are necessary for producing substances that are essential to the body (hormones, prostaglandins, and so on). The body is capable of storing fat in fat tissues as a sort of long-term energy reservoir. Excess consumption of fat (as well as all other foods containing calories) increases the fat reservoirs to virtually unlimited proportions. Fats can be of animal or vegetable origin.

Animal fats are found in butter, chicken skin, meat (beef, pork, poultry, and so on), and dairy products (creams, milk, yogurts, and cheeses). Excessive amounts of any of these foods containing animal fats make us put on weight and can damage our state of health by, for example, raising the cholesterol level in the blood and aiding in the development of cardiovascular and other diseases.

Vegetable fats are found mainly in liquid oils and margarine. It is important to note that, from a health-related point of view, I recommend olive or canola oil over oils such as safflower, sunflower, corn, etc. Olive and canola oils contain the largest portion of monounsaturated fat, the kind that helps reduce cholesterol and prevent diseases, such as cardiovascular disease and even certain cancers. Margarine (solid margarine in particular) and foods containing them (hydrogenated oils must be mentioned in the nutritional information on product packages) is not recommended because it contains trans fats that are now believed to be detrimental to your health.

You will spare yourself the torture of rigorous diets and self-starvation if you keep in mind that calories are not the enemy. They are actually friends because they give us life. The determining factor is how we balance their intake and expenditure. Unlike a bank account, where you are interested in saving, when it comes to your body account, you want to spend as much as you can.

ON THE BREAD FOR LIFE DIET it is not necessary to count calories because you eat small amounts of *complex* carbohydrates and other nutritious foods throughout the day. This helps you burn calories more efficiently and prevents you from overeating.

11

Sporty & Thin

Our ancient ancestors didn't have overweight or obesity problems. Although their lifestyle sounds monotonous compared to ours in the modern world, it was fraught with strenuous physical effort and oriented entirely toward survival. They ate little and irregularly. They wandered from place to place, looking for sources of food, water, and shelter. They obtained their meals by hunting animals and foraging for nuts, grains, and berries. Often they had to flee for their lives to escape hostile tribes or predators. In other words, they were very physically active.

The physiological and genetic foundations of the human race that enabled prehistoric people to eat little, survive long periods of famine between short periods of plenty, and to be physically active every day of their short lives have not changed during the thousands of years of human development. They are ingrained in us, like a master plan for the way we were expected to live.

The world in which we now live offers gratification of our whims at the click of the button. We could live almost our entire lives without moving from the couch. And we are fueling this inactivity with super-size meals. Food is there when we want it and in the amount we want. The wonders of modern existence have disturbed the balance between the amount of food we consume and the amount of physical activity we perform. Modern convenience is affecting our weight and our health.

THE BENEFITS OF EXERCISE

We all know that physical activity burns calories. Some of us are willing, able, and even eager to help restore balance after eating a cream-filled cake by speed walking for 2 hours or running for 1 hour. But not everyone is capable of handling such strenuous physical challenges.

So, what about everybody else? Here's the good news: Even moderate, regular physical activity, which most people can manage, is significantly beneficial because it helps promote weight loss and maintain physical and mental health. Most people can walk and can even ride a bicycle. A half-hour of either activity can burn about 150 to 200 calories, and indirectly burns more by revving up your metabolism.

There are two main types of physical activity:

Aerobic. This type includes any prolonged activity such as swimming or walking during which the muscles utilize oxygen to generate energy.

Anaerobic. This type includes short-term, very intense movements such as weight lifting, jumping, or sprinting short distances, during which the muscles do not depend on oxygen supply to produce energy.

Anaerobic exercise requires an intensity that few of us can muster and is generally not suitable for older people or very overweight or obese people. Aerobic is undoubtedly a better choice for most, at least in the beginning. Here are some of its advantages. It:

+ Burns calories.

+ Increases muscle mass and, consequently, increases basal metabolic rate, which contributes to weight loss.

+ Increases the activity of substances inside cells that are responsible for burning off energy. This contributes to a greater ability to burn calories, even for several hours after the exercise stops.

+ Improves mood, because it causes the secretion of endorphins (the body's natural painkillers and mood improvers) in the brain, and makes us alert and full of vitality.

+ Helps suppress appetite.

+ Strengthens the muscles, including the heart muscle.

+ Improves heart-lung tolerance, and consequently, can help prevent heart disease. Moreover, even if a person who regularly exercises has a heart attack, the chances are greater that the attack will be mild and the recovery more rapid. Studies indicate that even light physical activity, such as walking, gardening, or doing housework, exerts a positive effect in the prevention of heart disease, heart attacks, and strokes among men, and even more so among women.

This includes helping to:

+ Lower the blood levels of "bad" (LDL) cholesterol and raise the level of "good" (HDL) cholesterol.

+ Lower the blood level of triglycerides.

+ Lower the blood levels of sugar and insulin.

+ Reduce high blood pressure in many cases.

+ In addition, weight-bearing activities like walking and dancing helps improve bone density, thus helping to prevent osteoporosis.

One of the most recommended physical activities is walking. In addition to all the advantages listed above, it does not require special facilities or instructors, does not involve unnecessary expense (except for good walking shoes), and most people are capable of performing it at any age.

CALORIE-BURNING ACTIVITIES

Physical activity increases calorie burn, though not all of us burn calories at the same rate. Factors that make a difference are level of fitness (previous training), body composition (more fat, less expenditure; more muscle, more expenditure), age, gender, body weight, and, of course, genetics.

The table on page 155 will give you an idea of the average calories a person can expect to burn during different kinds of activities.

THE BEST EXERCISES FOR YOU

My recommendations regarding physical activity are walking or riding a bicycle, preferably outdoors. Most people who buy stationary exercise

CALORIE-BURNING ACTIVITIES

✦ ✦ ✦

Activity	Calories Burned		
(10 MIN.)	125 LBS.	175 LBS.	240 LBS.
Running (11.8 mph)	164	228	326
Climbing stairs	146	202	288
Running (5.6 mph)	90	125	178
Riding a bicycle (12.4 mph)	89	124	178
Playing tennis	56	80	115
Playing basketball	58	82	110
Walking (3.7 mph)	52	72	102
Aerobic dancing	48	66	94
Playing volleyball	43	65	94
Riding a bicycle (5.6 mph)	48	58	86
Swimming (crawl)	40	56	80
Scrubbing the floor	38	53	75
Square dancing	35	48	69
Cooking	32	46	65
Playing table tennis	32	45	64
Swimming (backstroke)	32	45	64
Nonstrenuous gardening	30	42	59
Walking (1.9 mph)	29	40	58
Dusting	22	31	44
Typing	19	27	39
Sitting	15	21	30
Standing	12	16	24
Sleeping	10	14	20
Watching television	10	14	18

bicycles for home use end up turning them into coat racks before long. I don't know why this happens, but I have found that hardly anyone actually uses them for longer than a couple of weeks. Think twice before spending your hard-earned money on such expensive exercise equipment.

Riding a road bike can be uncomfortable and scary for some people, but if you know how to maneuver traffic, it can be an enjoyable way to get exercise. Many cities now offer bicycle lanes on main streets to make riding safer and more enjoyable, and parks with bicycle paths are common.

Walking in the open air does not involve any expense and is not limited to defined time periods or special conditions, unless it rains or snows, of course, or the weather is especially hot. In such cases, you can walk indoors, for example, in a large mall. Walking does not require an instructor, though many clubs and groups have organized walks with instructors who lead people with varying skill levels on hikes and walks. Look for one in your town; it can be great fun.

Although many people enjoy swimming, walking offers a distinct advantage over it. Walking is a weight-bearing exercise (you use your muscles to hold up and move your own weight) and, therefore, contributes to improving bone density. It also helps suppress appetite (partly because it releases endorphins). This doesn't mean you shouldn't swim, but the water's buoyancy will keep you from getting all the benefits you would enjoy from a brisk hike. Besides, swimming often induces hunger. There are various theories about why this happens. One of them suggests that when we inevitably swallow pool water, the chlorine irritates our stomach lining, causing the impulse to eat.

Ideally, for weight loss, you should walk 45 minutes, five to seven times a week, but even 30 minutes will get the job done. Recent research shows that you can split your walking into 10- to 15-minute sessions a few times a day if you have difficulty walking longer. If you continue to walk on a regular basis, you will see significant results within a short time, and you won't want to give it up. You don't need to equip yourself with a pulse-monitor (heart-rate monitor) to force yourself to increase speed because every healthy person who continues to walk on a regular basis (down the street, around the park, or along the beach) will improve their heart-lung tolerance, develop their muscles, and naturally begin to move faster without any conscious intention.

Walking for 30 to 45 minutes five times a week is reasonable, convenient, and physiologically effective, but walking four times a week is better than not walking at all, and walking every day is better than five times a week. There are people who try to compensate for inactivity during the week by taking a strenuous 3-hour walk along a difficult route on the weekend. Sorry, but it doesn't work. This type of walking only tires the muscles and won't help you attain your goal.

If you walk on a treadmill, you can mechanically regulate your walking speed, but be careful: Some people increase it too much, and when they're finished, they can barely breathe or stay standing. If you walk on a treadmill at home or at a fitness club, it is important to know that you should not do so to the point of exhaustion. In fact, it likely will make you feel worse, not better. The goal is not to tire out your muscles, but to develop them. Too strenuous exercise, especially in nontrained people,

HATE EXERCISE?

Some people just won't exercise no matter what. Some try and quit. Some do their physical activity dutifully, only because they know it is good for them. Many grow to like it, and some even overdo it.

No matter what description fits you, *The Bread for Life Diet* works for your health, even without exercise. I recommend it because it is good for your health, and it also makes weight loss a lot easier.

FITNESS CLUBS

If you can afford the membership fee, a gym or fitness club can offer an excellent environment for exercise, provided you know how to work out or the club offers trained instructors to guide you. Without proper training, you could push your body beyond its capability and end up discouraged or even cause an injury. Proper training, in addition to being safe, will help make for a pleasant experience.

Also, beware of nutritional advice from club employees. They often are not professional nutritionists and can mislead you with wrong information. Make sure that they are not trying to sell you some product that the club offers. Fortunately, in recent years, many fitness clubs have begun employing registered dietitians to advise their clients, and that is a benefit you can comfortably take advantage of.

can cause soreness in the muscles and joints, tear ligaments, and can even be harmful to the heart.

Increase the intensity and speed gradually so that you give your muscles time to adapt to the brisker pace. When you walk without a treadmill, you usually do not get exhausted because there is no artificial factor increasing your speed. You move according to your ability and desire.

Keep in mind that any kind of physical activity is beneficial and will help you reach your goals. For example, gardening, other yard work, and house work are good exercise. Fast dancing and square dancing are fun ways to stay active. Also, you can always park your car a distance from your destination and walk. Take the stairs instead of the elevator, but for no more than three or four floors. If you must reach a higher floor, get off a few flights below your destination and take the stairs.

Dogs are great motivators for getting you out and walking several times a day. Plus, they make a loyal friend and walking companion.

NOT RECOMMENDED

Running is an excellent activity for people who are fit enough to do it. But it is not recommended for people who are overweight and looking for a way to get into exercise. It burns more calories than walking, but otherwise the advantages are similar. Overweight people often just are not active or supple enough to choose running. Besides, overweight people are more prone to damaging their knee and hip joints when running. Neither is it a good idea for older people to begin running (or to participate in a sport that requires intense running, such as tennis) without consulting a health professional.

In general, before performing any physical activity, unfit or older people should always seek professional advice. Studies indicate that there is a danger of heart attack, not to mention of orthopedic injuries, among untrained people who begin strenuous and difficult activities without proper preparation.

Avoid activities that stress the knees and hip joints because, in the long run, they can cause damage. For example, do not walk or run up or down steep hills, climb or descend more than three or four flights of steps at a time, and avoid using a stair-climbing machine for exercise.

The recommendation is that you exercise moderately. Setting a level of performance that is too high will cause more problems than it solves, sometimes even irreversible ones.

A GOOD ATTITUDE AND GOOD SHOES

In order to make physical activity a real part of your lifestyle, especially at first, it's better to pick something you enjoy but it must also be beneficial. What was the first thought that came to mind when you started reading this chapter? "Oh, no! Must I exercise?"

The answer is that you don't *have to*, but it would be very beneficial for you. Forget the excuse that it is too hard and too exhausting, and yes, boring. This only happens in the beginning. It gets easier. Deep down you understand it is important, so change your negative thoughts to positive ones: "It's fun, effective, and enjoyable, and it's worthwhile for me to do it."

I have a tip that might help. Sing as you walk. It will help you to mentally relax. Why? Because when you focus on the words you are singing you cannot think, and when you're not thinking, stress tends to melt away.

When you walk, it's very important to wear shoes that fit well, are comfortable, and are in good condition. Taking care of your body also means taking care of your feet, since they are meant to carry you through the rest of your life. Do not walk wearing worn-out shoes, and don't wear ordinary sneakers, either. Wear socks that don't cause your feet to perspire and do not crowd your foot in the shoe.

THE BREAD FOR LIFE DIET, combined with physical activity, enables you to burn off calories and increase energy expenditure, thereby promoting weight loss, a significant reduction in body measurements, and overall improved health.

12

An Odd Array of Diets

When it comes to topics of conversation, diets and dieting are right up there with politics and the weather. It's no wonder. On any given day, one in every six people is following some kind of diet. Among teenage girls, it is even more. Statistics indicate that approximately two-thirds of female high-school students in the United States are involved in some kind of weight-loss program.

There is no shortage of diets from which to choose. Pick any program, follow it precisely. and, more often than not, you will lose weight, and just as likely, you will gain it back. That's because most people view losing weight as the end of the road. In reality, it is just the beginning.

Yes, it would be great to go on a diet, reach your weight-loss goal, and never have to worry about dieting again. Unfortunately, it doesn't work this way. If you want to reach and maintain your target weight, you may want to abandon the illusion that you'll wake up thin one day and be thin every day after that. I call this dream diet the "Abracadabra Illusion Diet"—it has yet to be invented. To maintain the weight you want, you have to adopt a diet—that is, an eating style—that becomes a permanent way of life.

Few people can follow a diet that seems like a list of prohibitions and restrictions for very long. On the other hand, it is very possible to follow an eating style even for life when it is perceived as a good habit and a satisfying way of living.

If you are reading this book, chances are you have tried some type of diet before. Perhaps, over the course of your life, you have tried several different diets, some of which yielded better results than others. Each time, after the diet "ended," you started heading back up to your old weight. Then back to yet another diet.

This kind of diet behavior is quite common. Unfortunately, it is a vicious cycle because it frequently means that after each new diet, you end up weighing more than you did before you started the diet. How frustrating! I call this kind of weight gain "diet-induced obesity." When I ask a patient on our first meeting what diets he or she had been on, some of them say: "Oh, you name it, there is no diet I haven't tried. You are my last hope!" or "If I had known what weight I'd reach, I would never have started any diet at all and be much thinner." The interesting thing is that the more diets they've tried, the more overweight they are.

Yes, there are a lot of diets out there that work. The problem is, they only work as long as people stick to the program. Once the diet is "over," the weight comes back. A lot of people go off a diet even before they reach their weight-loss goal. The reason? Most diets are not very sustainable.

YO-YO DIETS AND RODENTS

The gain-lose-gain cycle known as yo-yo dieting has been studied extensively by laboratory researchers. In one experiment, rodents were given a low-calorie diet alternated with a high-calorie diet. They repeatedly gained and lost weight, but the rate at which they gained and lost weight changed with each cycle. During the first round of being fed a low-calorie diet, weight loss lasted 21 days. When the newly thin rodents were then put on a normal diet, it took them 46 days to get back to their original weight. During the second round, however, it took the rodents 56 days to lose weight, and only 24 days to return to their original weight.

This experiment demonstrates that there is a *physiological* basis for the phenomena produced by the yo-yo diet, as rodents are not affected by mental factors, moods, boredom, and all the other causes that we customarily cite as excuses for weight gain among humans.

LOW- AND VERY-LOW-CALORIE DIETS

The most popular diets, especially among young people, are low-calorie ones. It makes perfect sense to people that the less they eat, the more weight they will lose. True—but only in the short term. Eventually, if they manage to stick with it, they discover at some point that the less they eat, the less they lose. That's because decreasing calories is a sure way to slow down your metabolism. The body is programmed just as it was in our hunter-gatherer days to conserve calories (by reducing the energy burn rate so it can hang on to every calorie as long as possible) in case of a possible food shortage. This is the reason why many people who go on a low-calorie diet eventually stop losing weight or even gain a couple of pounds despite continued dieting. When they start adding more food to their diets, even a small amount, an immediate weight gain follows.

The moment you decide to radically reduce the amount of food you consume, you are actually making a decision to gain weight—and in an unhealthy way. With each weight loss, the body breaks down muscle tissue in addition to fat tissue; when you regain weight, mostly fat tissue is rebuilt. So it is not your imagination: You really do get fatter. You have increased the percentage of your body fat.

Many of my patients have been victims of this weight-loss/weight-gain syndrome commonly called yo-yo dieting. They were horrified to discover that the more they restricted their food intake—for some as little as 500 to 600 calories a day—the worse the eventual outcome after they got back to "normal" eating. "How is it possible? What do I do now?" they ask.

I tell them that they need to eat more, not less, in order to lose weight and keep it off. When I put them on *The Bread for Life Diet*, they respond with concern. "So much food? I'll get fat!" Then, to their great surprise, they lose weight. But this is the way the body was designed to work. The right number of calories encourages a normal, faster metabolism.

It is essential to remember that at one point or another in every diet, even *The Bread for Life Diet*, weight loss will halt, but only temporarily. This is a signal that your body has stabilized to a new metabolic state. The professional term for this state is "plateau." In everyday language, it simply means "getting stuck." If you continue with your diet, you can reasonably assume that your weight will resume dropping, and then, at some point, will stabilize again. After each plateau, the next one will usually come sooner and last longer because the body becomes more and more efficient at adapting its metabolism to the calories you supply (or don't supply) it. It learns from experience.

Low-calorie (less than 1,000 calories a day) and very-low-calorie (less than 600 calories a day) diets, when followed for more than a few days, can be harmful to your health. Severe calorie restriction can cause symptoms such as dehydration, a sharp drop in blood pressure and blood sugar levels, nausea, headaches, hair loss, constipation, an unpleasant taste in the mouth, bad breath, vitamin and mineral imbalance, fatigue, a sensation of cold, and muscle pain. Women in particular report bad moods, insomnia, and even depression. Severe calorie restriction can also lead to a halt in the menstrual cycle and can lead to anorexia, a life-threatening eating disorder.

HIGH-PROTEIN DIETS

High-protein diets, also known as low-carbohydrate diets, are simple to follow because the amounts are usually generous and your food choices are limited, consisting primarily of meat, eggs, and high-fat dairy products, such as cheese, sour cream, butter, and cream. Weight loss is usually fast at the beginning, and after a few days, you even feel less hungry.

On the surface, this seems like a perfect recipe, but it is only effective in the short term. Long term, it has no superior qualities over other diets and can even be harmful. The brain, nervous system, blood cells, and, to a lesser extent, kidneys depend on carbohydrates to function. In the absence of carbohydrates in the diet, the body is forced to produce glucose by breaking down the body's proteins—that is, the muscles. This causes the body to excrete a considerable amount of water, which is why people who are on protein diets report going to the bathroom many times both during the day and at night.

Uric acid, one of the products of the breakdown of proteins, is liable to accumulate and settle in the joints of the hands and feet, causing gout (a form of arthritis) in sensitive people. In addition, excess protein, together with a lack of carbohydrates, causes a sharp drop in the level of serotonin. As you now know, this causes cravings for sweets. It also causes bad moods, irritability, nervousness, lack of focus and loss of energy. Women, who naturally have lower serotonin levels than men, usually find it harder to maintain a protein diet for long periods of time.

Most people who go on this type of diet do not persevere over time because of the monotony of eating nothing but protein. The craving for carbohydrates usually causes them to break the diet sooner or later. It is essential to drink plenty of fluids while on a protein diet, as the increased fluid excretion can lead to dehydration. Another reason is that protein diets cause the accumulation of protein breakdown by-products in the blood, which overburdens the kidneys.

The Complete Scarsdale Medical Diet, The Zone Diet, and *The South Beach Diet* are all high-protein, carbohydrate-restricted diets with a few modifications that make them slightly different from each other. These deviations involve the number and kinds of vegetables and carbohydrates allowed at various stages.

Dr. Atkins New Diet Revolution is similar to these diets but puts more emphasis on fat-rich proteins. People adjust to it more easily, because it consists of tastier food, such as cheese with high fat content and juicy steaks in unlimited amounts. However, it is open to all the side effects associated with other protein diets with one addition: It can speed up the process of arteriosclerosis (hardening of the arteries) because of its high content of saturated fat and cholesterol.

MONO DIETS

"Mono" diets mean eating is restricted to a single type of food (e.g., potatoes, meat, bananas, or rice) each day, according to a predetermined order. The extreme lack of variety naturally causes the dieter to reduce the amount of food consumed, and therefore, to lose weight.

One of the more recent mono diets that got a lot of fanfare was the cabbage soup diet. The soup is permitted in unlimited quantities, is filling, tasty, and provides fluids and fiber. But how long can you eat the same kind of soup? And who wants to be eating soup during the hot summer?

The extreme nature of the diet and the need for special preparation (making the soup, having soup available wherever you go) makes it difficult to adhere to and difficult to maintain as part of one's daily routine.

COMBINATION DIETS

This type of diet restricts mixing proteins and carbohydrates at the same meal. This principle has no basis in human physiology. Health-wise, it's perfectly okay to eat proteins and carbohydrates together with no resulting damage whatsoever. Think about milk (dairy or breast or infant formula). It's often the only food babies are fed, and it supplies all the necessary nutrients they need—protein, fat, and carbohydrates. Legumes also contain proteins and carbohydrates, and even carbohydrate-rich foods like bread and potatoes contain a small amount of protein. In fact, most foods contain some amount of both protein and carbohydrates, because this combination occurs in nature, and the body knows how to handle it perfectly.

Combination diets do have a positive effect, since meals within the framework of this kind of diet tend to be monotonous, so you naturally reduce the amount of food you eat. A meal composed of meat and potatoes is generally larger than a meal composed of only meat or only potatoes. How much meat can you eat? How many mashed potatoes can you stuff yourself with? Restriction causes eating smaller meals, which we already know helps in losing weight.

The disadvantage of the combination diet lies mainly in the fact that it is low in bread and grains, milk and meat, which provide protein, fats, vitamins, and important minerals.

THE BLOOD TYPE DIET

This diet, with its unique spin, quickly became a best seller. The book, entitled *Eat Right For Your Type*, is fascinating even though it is not based on scientific evidence. The diet works the way any diet would work if you believe in it and follow it rigorously. The book proposes four types of diets according to the four blood types. All of them are low in fat and sugar, with certain differences in the amounts of dairy products, meat, bread, vegetables, and fruit. Obviously, the dieter will lose weight. Overall, the diet is fairly balanced.

FORMULA (LIQUID) DIETS

These diets are based on drinking beverages made from powders. If the formula is your only source of nutrition, the dangers are the same as in low-calorie diets. Because of reports of damage to health, including cases of death, the companies that manufacture formulas recommend eating two regular meals and only one formula meal a day. Drinking the powdered beverage only once a day is not harmful, but the 200 to 300 calories that it provides can be obtained from ordinary food (four slices of light bread with a spread, or chicken breast with salad, for example), which is both tastier, less expensive, and more filling. Liquids, no matter how thick, don't do as much to make you feel satisfied. Even though these formulas are fortified with nutrients, it doesn't make them healthy.

JUICE DIETS

A variety of juice diets have come in and out of fashion. They are the classic definition of a fad diet! Essentially, they are based solely on drinking water as well as natural fruit and vegetable juices in the "name of health." Their self-proclaimed goal is to cleanse the body, but in principle our bodies are built to "cleanse" themselves. The body is equipped with all the necessary "cleansing" systems it needs, including the blood and lymphatic systems, the digestive system, the kidneys and urinary system, the respiratory system, and perspiration and other secretions.

With regard to weight loss, people who drink only water and juice for a period of a few days increase their chance of losing weight, but there are people for whom drinking fruit juice, which contains sugar, causes a halt in the weight-loss process. Most of the food groups are missing from this kind of diet, and over time it is liable to cause health problems, such as disruptions of the body's mineral balance, diarrhea, dizziness, and weakness.

WEIGHT WATCHERS

This is a nutritionally balanced diet that was designed for the long haul and to become a way of life. It is suitable for healthy people who want to maintain their weight and don't mind being weighed every week in a group setting. Many people say that participating in the group setting provides positive reinforcement. However, the groups receive instruction from participants who have lost weight rather than by health professionals possessing in-depth knowledge of nutrition and the ability to identify health problems.

OTHER WAYS OF LOSING WEIGHT

Some people, mostly those who have tried and failed, will go to extremes in an effort to lose weight. Some methods can be helpful, but some are downright dangerous. So beware!

Diuretics. Taking water pills causes the body to excrete fluid by urinating in extreme volume. That makes you lower your weight superficially because you are losing water but not burning up any fat tissue. The use of diuretics poses health risks, whether the diuretics are natural or if they are chemically made. Even if a label says "natural," it is not a guarantee that the product is good for your health. Natural is not a synonym for healthy!

Laxatives. The use of laxatives can cause superficial weight loss, which again is due to the loss of fluids and in no way to the breakdown of fat. Using laxatives for losing weight is popular among women, and young women in particular. They often claim that they are trying to cleanse their bodies, but as explained above, the body does this on its own. Taking laxatives on a prolonged basis can cause the loss of fluids and minerals, dehydration, weakness, headaches, fainting, and even damage to the mucous membrane of the colon. Excessive use of laxatives is also liable to lead to dependence on the laxative for the bowels to function normally.

Acupuncture. This can aid in weight loss, not because it suppresses appetite, but because it can relieve some of the discomforts that give rise to uncontrolled eating, such as irritability and headaches. Unfortunately, some therapists prescribe rigorous diets along with acupuncture. If you opt for acupuncture, take dietary advice only from a qualified nutritional expert, dietitian, or doctor.

Medications. Diet pills can work but they are generally recommended only for people who are obese and must lose weight to regain their health. There are two types of medicines that work in two different ways. Those that affect the brain's serotonin and norepinephrine levels (Meridia™, for example) help to suppress appetite and do an excellent job at it—for a little while. They also have side effects that are hard for some people to tolerate, such as headaches, sleeping problems, dry mouth, and an increase in blood pressure.

Medicines that affect the digestive system and reduce the absorption of fat from food (Xenical™) also pose possible side effects, including gas and diarrhea. These medicines are all prescription and should be taken only under the supervision of a qualified doctor.

Fasting. Eliminating all food is not a particularly healthful or effective way to lose weight. During a fast, people lose mainly muscle mass and fluids. Fasting for a day or two is not harmful for a healthy person. On the other hand, long fasts cause all the same problems that come with low-calorie diets and juice diets, only with more severe consequences.

Weight-loss spas or fat farms. Going off for a week or two to indulge in gourmet low-fat meals, exercise, and leisure-time pampering is an enjoyable way to lose weight for people who have the time and money to take advantage of them. They sound great, but guess what happens when you leave paradise and return to the daily grind? Yes, you guessed it! The magic wears off and the weight comes back.

Gastric surgery. Although there are different types of surgery, all are an extreme means of getting rid of fat and should be limited to people who suffer from morbid obesity (a BMI of over 30), which constitutes a danger to health. Different types of gastric surgery physically reduce the amount of food that can enter the stomach. However, surgery does not alter the mind, which still makes it possible, even after the surgery, to gobble down enough chocolate and milkshakes to put the weight back on. Unfortunately, that happens all too often after such a surgery. Also, because it is a surgical procedure, it carries its share of health risks.

Liposuction. This type of surgery is used mainly to repair aesthetic flaws, that is, to "improve" the appearance of the body. It has been shown that liposuction in the upper belly, however, does not reduce the health risks of the apple-shape obesity.

Gadgets. Contraptions for weight loss are constantly advertised in the media. These include various kinds of belts, creams that "dissolve" fat, electrodes, special pants, various types of "effortless" exercise, and pills that guarantee you'll lose weight with no dieting or physical activity. There is a lot of suspicion as to their ability to live up to their claims. Think twice before spending your money on any of these.

THE BREAD FOR LIFE DIET is a sensible and healthy diet that permits you to eat sanely, and enjoy delicious food without ever feeling hungry as you lose weight. It is a diet that can be maintained so you can sustain your weight loss and never gain weight again.

13

Secrets of Success

Whether you are going on *The Bread for Life Diet* to lose weight, retain your weight, or improve your health, adapting to a new eating style can get a little rocky from time to time. I have a few tips that I hope you will find helpful when confronted with some of the issues. I've also addressed some all-too-common myths that are popular among dieters. These myths are rooted in unreliable information that gets passed around and even ends up in the media. The Frequently Asked Questions are the most common queries I receive from patients at my weight loss clinic. Hopefully, they will answer all your questions, too.

TIP: IDENTIFY AND CONFRONT OVEREATING

This is not always as easy as it sounds because at least some of your overeating habits may seem "normal" to you.

For example, you stop by the bakery every Friday, because it has become a treat that your family looks forward to. Only thing is you always get extra and end up eating more than anyone else once you get home. If you step back and think through a routine that is negatively affecting your weight-loss efforts, it can help you identify the issues and determine what changes to make. Here is the sample step-by-step description for the bakery scenario above:

I buy the pastries every week; I buy the pastries at the same shop every time; I buy pastries for everyone, plus some; I always put the bag on the kitchen counter; I settle in for an evening of watching television and before long, I feel like eating something; I go to the kitchen where I "find" the pastries on the counter (what a surprise); I take one, then decide to grab a few instead and head back to the TV; I enjoy the first few bites but before I know it, they are all gone; I feel guilty and like I've blown my eating plan for the whole week; I eat the whole bag.

Identifying and understanding each aspect of the problem makes it possible for you to be aware of the cycle and to stop it at any stage. You can decide to buy pastries less often, avoid the bakery, buy fewer pastries, put the bag in an inconspicuous place, eat only half a pastry, or choose a different snack like popcorn (without butter) instead.

Identify every situation that causes you to overeat. Being aware of these situations enables you to prepare yourself for them, so that you can control them and prevent them from controlling you.

FREQUENTLY ASKED QUESTION

"Is *The Bread for Life Diet* as good for someone who wants to lose 5 to 10 pounds as it is for someone who wants to lose 60 pounds?"
In principle, yes, but people who want to lose 5 pounds don't usually need a diet. It is usually enough for them to eat fewer sweet and fattening foods. They can also go on *The Bread for Life Diet* starting directly at Stage Two.

TIP: KEEP A FOOD LIST

Keeping a food diary really does make dieting easier for you. I often recommend this technique to my patients. It means they must make a list of each and every food or drink as soon as it goes into their mouths (not later when they have a chance to "forget"). Patients often come back to me a week later a few pounds lighter, even before I have given them their dieting instructions. Why? Because writing it down made them aware of what and how much they ate.

We tend to forget what we eat. For example, we don't take notice of grazing, especially when it comes to "small" treats, like a few nuts or a few pretzels. Often, it is the foods you don't remember consuming that are the ones that cause you to put on weight. So when you eat something— even if you have taken just a taste while cooking—write it down. No need to calculate calories or even amounts. Just write it down. You'll be surprised at how much you decide not to put in your mouth when you realize that you have to pick up your pencil and add it to your list!

FREQUENTLY ASKED QUESTION

"Does it matter what kind of bread you eat—white or whole-grain?"
Whole-grain bread is more healthful because of its lower glycemic index and high fiber content, but eating white bread once in a while does no harm.

TIP: FIND WAYS TO SOCIALIZE THAT DON'T INCLUDE EATING

When people get together for business or pleasure, it is often over a meal. Think of alternatives, such as walking together, drinking coffee (without cake), or going shopping. On those occasions when a get-together does involve a meal, select a place that is known for its salads, omelets, or soups, instead of a bakery that is famous for its cakes piled high with whipped cream and frosting.

"Why is there no calorie counting on The Bread for Life Diet?"

When you're on *The Bread for Life Diet*, you don't need to count calories because eating carbohydrates prevents hunger attacks and eating frenzies, thereby making calorie counting unnecessary. If you're not hungry, you don't overeat. For many people, counting calories is compulsive.

One hundred calories, more or less, is not what makes people gain weight. Uncontrolled eating does, because it increases intake by several hundred calories at a time. On the other hand, when you eat filling food every 3 to 4 hours, the need to count calories disappears.

TIP: EAT BEFORE YOU GET THERE

If you're going to an event that will offer an abundance of fattening and delicious food, make sure that you do not arrive hungry. My patients who have adopted this rule tell me that this technique helps them be more selective about their choices and more in control of their eating.

A good tactic, especially when confronted with a buffet, is to start with a few diet drinks or glasses of water first. Then always go for the less-fattening foods first, such as salads, a roll, small sandwiches, and even fruit. It leaves less room on your plate when you hit the section that contains the main dishes that most likely add the largest number of calories. Ignore the dessert table altogether! Remind yourself that you can always come back for more later. Chances are you won't take that second trip.

TIP: MAKE UP YOUR OWN MIND

When dining in restaurants, ignore what other people at the table are ordering. Once you decide what's best for you to order, close the menu and stick to your choice regardless of what others at the table order. If you are easily influenced by everyone else's choices, ask to order first. There is nothing wrong with tasting what the other diners are having, but keep it to just a taste.

TIP: LIMIT TEMPTATIONS AT HOME

We are all familiar with the excuses, "I buy cookies for the children" or "I keep pastries in the freezer for guests." People often confess to me, however, that the children don't necessarily like those kinds of cookies or that guests come by only once a month. Think of the extent to which we are prepared to believe our own excuses, and then let go of them. There is a proverb that goes, "Do not bring enemies into your home." Make it happen.

MYTH: EATING BETWEEN MEALS IS FORBIDDEN.

Just the opposite is true: Not eating between meals is forbidden. People who eat frequent and small meals store less fat than those who eat one or two large meals a day. They also have fewer cravings for sweets.

TIP: USE SMART SHOPPING STRATEGIES

There are two main rules for buying food: First, do your shopping when you're full so that hunger doesn't influence you to buy foods that are unnecessary and fattening. Second, go shopping with a detailed list of all the groceries that you need and don't let yourself be tempted into buying unnecessary foods on impulse.

Also, when you are food shopping, don't succumb to the temptation to buy big economy-size packages, especially when it comes to treats like cookies, pretzels, and nuts. Saving a little money is no substitute for the temptation it brings to you and also your family.

"Is the diet suitable for diabetics?"

This diet is suitable for people with type 2 diabetes who do not receive insulin. The current medical recommendations for them are: spread out small meals over the day (every 3 to 4 hours), eat a complex carbohydrate content of 45 to 65 percent of total calorie intake, and lose excess weight. All these are the foundations of *The Bread for Life Diet*.

Diabetics who receive insulin injections are not included in this category; they need a diet designed by a registered dietitian.

TIP: TAKE A 20-MINUTE PAUSE

If you suddenly feel the urge to eat something you know you shouldn't be eating, look at the clock and wait 20 minutes. Most likely, you are bored rather than hungry. The food will still be there after 20 minutes, but you'll have enough time to cancel the "sudden and immediate" stimulus in your brain, helping you overcome the urge to eat. If after 20 minutes you still decide to eat whatever it is you feel like eating, go for it. This rule is also applicable if you still feel hungry after a meal.

MYTH: BODY WEIGHT DEPENDS ONLY ON THE NUMBER OF CALORIES YOU EAT.

Wrong. Body weight is greatly determined by metabolic and genetic mechanisms. This means that two people can eat the same amount of calories and do the same amount of exercise, but one can still be fatter than the other, depending upon how economical their bodies are at storing fat.

TIP: DON'T WATCH AND EAT AT THE SAME TIME

A lot of people like to eat while watching television or reading a newspaper or a book. By doing this, we put food in our mouths without noticing and "forget" what and how much we're eating. Some practical advice: Find an alternative activity while watching television or reading. For example, give yourself a manicure, knit, or squeeze a hand grip strengthener or a tennis ball. Anything that keeps your fingers busy and prevents you from reaching for food will do.

MYTH: THE BEST WAY TO CUT CALORIES IS TO SKIP MEALS.

People who skip meals in order to eat fewer calories are actually setting themselves up for excessive eating, primarily in the afternoon and evening. Skipping meals means that you will inevitably end up more hungry. You'll feel famished. When you are this hungry, your resistance to food is at its lowest and it becomes hard to keep yourself from eating whatever is in sight. Eating too much will agitate your insulin level and send your blood sugar on a roller-coaster ride.

TIP: LEARN TO SAY "NO, THANK YOU"

Saying "No, thank you" politely and with determination is not insulting. Think about it. If you had diabetes, no host would try to persuade you to eat cake. On the other hand, when people say, "I'm on a diet," sometimes a host will nag you even more, saying things like, "Not today," or "Not in my house." Be firm. If necessary, say that you eat only healthy foods. That will generally take the wind out of their sails.

MYTH: A SWEET APPLE IS MORE FATTENING THAN A SOUR ONE.

In reality, both kinds have the same number of calories per ounce. The bigger they are, the more calories they contain. Choose whichever apple you prefer, and the smaller the better.

TIP: DON'T USE FOOD FOR COMFORT

Since we all know that eating is related to emotions, come up with alternative ways to deal with your feelings that don't involve eating. Consider other little treats, such as taking a bubble bath, chatting on the phone with a friend, going on a shopping spree, having a facial or a body massage, meditating, or, better yet, going outdoors and getting some exercise. Everyone is entitled to get in a bad mood from time to time. It's perfectly normal. Just don't use food to comfort yourself.

MYTH: DRINKING WATER WITH A MEAL IS UNHEALTHY.

It is healthy and highly recommended to drink liquids before, during, and after meals, as well as between meals. It doesn't dilute digestive juices, as some people claim. Drink seven to nine 8-ounce glasses a day. Any kind of liquid is fine as long as it does not contain sugar or alcohol, as these substances are not substitutes for replenishing liquids.

TIP: PUT UP A STOP SIGN

Write the word "STOP" in large letters on a piece of paper and put it on the door of the refrigerator. It will make you think twice when you're standing in front of the door, and might even prevent you from opening it.

> ## MYTH: AVOIDING BREAD AND OTHER CARBOHY-DRATES WILL MAKE YOU LOSE WEIGHT.
>
> Bread and carbohydrates are of considerable importance to the human body because they are the brain's main fuel source. Abstaining from eating bread and other complex carbohydrates or opposing the demands of the body in any other way will elicit an unwelcome reaction—an increased and uncontrolled demand for carbohydrates in the form of sweets. The body requires all components of food: protein, carbohydrates, and even fats. *The Bread for Life Diet* is designed to give you the right amount of each for both weight control and health.

TIP: DON'T NIBBLE WHILE YOU COOK

Pay attention to situations in which you eat extra food without noticing or even without enjoying it. Perhaps you like eating broken pieces of cookies, "tasting" while you are cooking, or "straightening the corners" on a cake. Snacking this way can add a lot of extra calories to your daily food consumption.

When you "straighten the corners" on a cake or eat broken cookies, you end up eating much more, definitely enjoying it less, and gaining weight.

"Is the diet suitable for people with high cholesterol, elevated triglycerides, or high blood pressure?"

The Bread for Life Diet is suitable for people with high cholesterol because it is low in cholesterol and animal fats and contains vegetable fats, and for people with high triglycerides because it is low in sugar, alcohol, and fruit. Many people who have followed *The Bread for Life Diet* have experienced a significant drop in sugar, cholesterol, and triglyceride levels in their blood.

People who have high blood pressure also have experienced a drop in blood pressure thanks to *The Bread for Life Diet*. First, it helps because the drop in weight over time aids in stabilizing blood pressure for most people. Second, the diet contains vegetables, whole grains, and vegetable fat. People with high blood pressure should limit their salt intake.

TIP: DON'T GIVE UP ON EXERCISE

Here's why:

+ It makes you constantly aware of being on the health track.

+ It makes staying with your diet easier.

+ It makes your waist thinner.

+ It tones your muscles.

+ It improves your mood.

+ It makes you feel great about what you have accomplished.

These are all very important motivators for staying with your diet. Be active, be in motion.

However, even if you do not exercise, or exercised and quit, this does not mean you should quit dieting. *The Bread for Life Diet* works, even without exercising. You just won't experience its full potential.

FREQUENTLY ASKED QUESTION

"Does everybody lose weight at a similar speed?"

The speed at which people lose weight varies from one person to another, and decreases with age. It is also slower among women than among men, but this is true of weight loss in general. Some people will easily lose 5 pounds in a week, and for others it may take several weeks. Each person has to come to terms with the speed at which they lose weight. Some people will need to lower their expectations to avoid feeling disappointed.

Remember, how much weight you lose doesn't matter; what matters is that you do lose weight. No matter how desperately you want to become instantly svelte, weight loss depends on the unique features of your body, not only on your willpower. Remember that the result of not losing weight quickly enough is frustration, which leads to giving up, and regaining the weight already lost. So don't rush, take it easy, and let your body do the job as efficiently and thoroughly as it can.

14

Bread for Life Recipes

Simplicity is one of the keys to the ease of *The Bread for Life Diet*, and that applies to these recipes, which I call "recipes for those who don't like to cook." Those who enjoy cooking can, of course, modify or adjust the recipes according to their fancy, as long as they remain consistent with the rules and principles of the diet. Some of the dishes can be eaten in unlimited amounts and others can be used as bread substitutes.

Enjoy!

MAIN DISHES ➤

Green Fettuccine with Roasted Vegetables

Each serving of this dish can be counted as two slices of light bread.

1 pound green fettuccine

3 bell peppers, cut into strips (use different colors, if desired)

1 eggplant, diced

2 zucchini, sliced

6 garlic cloves, crushed

3 tablespoons olive oil

Salt and black pepper to taste

½ pound feta cheese (up to 5% fat)

1 ounce basil leaves, chopped

Preheat the oven to 425°F.

Prepare the fettuccine according to the instructions on the package.

Arrange the vegetables, and the garlic, in a pan (8" x 12" rectangular or 11" round), in rows, in a flat and uniform layer. Brush the vegetables lightly with the olive oil and sprinkle with salt and pepper.

Roast the vegetables in the oven for a very short time. Make sure the vegetables don't get too soft.

Transfer the vegetables into a large skillet or wok, add the cooked fettuccine, and stir while heating.

Add the cheese and basil and serve hot.

Serves 6

Pasta and Sun-Dried-Tomato Salad

Each serving of this pasta salad can be counted as two slices of light bread.

1 pound ziti, rigatoni, or penne pasta

1 small jar sun-dried tomatoes in olive oil, drained and cut into strips

1 ounce basil leaves, chopped

4-5 garlic cloves, sliced

2-3 tablespoons pine nuts, lightly toasted

Prepare the pasta according to the instructions on the package.

In a large bowl, mix the remaining ingredients. Add the cooked pasta and stir.

Let stand for a few hours. Serve at room temperature.

Serves 6

Rice Salad

Each serving can be counted as two slices of light bread.

3 cups water

1 cup basmati rice or brown rice

3 spring onions, chopped

2 tablespoons olive oil

2 bell peppers, diced (use different colors, if desired)

2 tablespoons freshly squeezed lemon juice

1 tomato, diced

¼ cup chopped parsley

Salt and black pepper to taste

Boil the water in a large saucepan. Add the rice and cook until soft. Drain and rinse in cold water.

Add the remaining ingredients. Stir until well-mixed. Chill before serving.

Serves 4

Chinese Vegetable Stir-Fry

Stir-fries can be very inventive and you can add different vegetables. The dish can be eaten in unlimited amounts. You can add chicken or seafood and eat it as a protein meal. Alternatively, you can add ⅔ cup of cooked rice or pasta and eat it as a substitute for two slices of bread.

Sauce:

½ cup water

⅓ cup soy sauce

Artificial sweetener
(equivalent of 2 tablespoons sugar)

4 garlic cloves, crushed

Stir-Fry:

2 tablespoons canola oil

1 medium onion, sliced

6 celery stalks,
cut into 1" pieces

6 spring onions,
cut into 1" pieces

2 red bell peppers, cut in narrow slices

2 cups small cauliflower florets

½ pound mushrooms, chopped

Grated ginger to taste

Prepare the sauce in a small bowl by mixing the water, soy sauce, sweetener, and garlic. Set aside.

Heat a wok or large frying pan and add the canola oil.

Add the onion, celery, spring onions, peppers, and cauliflower and stir-fry for 5 minutes.

Pour the sauce on the vegetables and stir-fry for 5 more minutes.

Add the mushrooms and ginger and continue to stir-fry for another 5 minutes.

Serves 4

Barley and Vegetable Casserole

This filling casserole can be a meal in itself! Each serving counts as two slices of light bread.

3 tablespoons olive oil

½ pound barley

1 small eggplant, finely diced

Salt and black pepper to taste

1 small onion, diced

1 small cauliflower, separated into florets

1 cup green beans, sliced

¼ cup chopped fresh oregano, for garnish

Preheat the oven to 400°F.

In a large pot, heat 1 tablespoon of the oil and fry the barley for a few minutes. Add water to cover the barley by about 6 inches. Cover and cook for approximately 1 hour until the barley is soft. Drain and set aside.

Toss the eggplant with 1 tablespoon of olive oil and sprinkle the pieces with salt and pepper. Place on a baking sheet and bake for approximately 10 minutes, or until soft.

In a large pot, heat the remaining tablespoon of oil and add the onion, cauliflower, and beans, and cook over high heat for 5 minutes. Cover, lower the heat, and steam for approximately 15 minutes until the vegetables are soft (add water as necessary).

Add the barley and eggplant to the vegetables and stir gently. Season with salt and pepper, garnish with fresh oregano, and serve.

Serves 6

Beet Leaf and Chick-Pea Casserole

Each serving can be counted as two slices of light bread.

¼ pound chick-peas

2 tablespoons olive oil

1 medium onion, chopped

3–4 garlic cloves, crushed

1 pound beet leaves or Swiss chard leaves, chopped

½ ounce coriander or parsley, chopped

Salt, to taste

1 teaspoon freshly squeezed lemon juice

½ teaspoon turmeric (optional)

Soak the dried chick-peas in water overnight. Pour off the water and add 1 quart of fresh water. Cook until soft. Strain and set aside.

In a heavy pot, heat the oil and sauté the onion, garlic, and beet leaves or Swiss chard leaves for approximately 10 minutes, until soft. Add a small amount of water, if necessary, and cover the pot.

Add the chick-peas and steam for approximately 10 more minutes.

Stir in the coriander or parsley, salt, lemon juice, and turmeric, if using. Cook for 5 minutes more and serve.

Serves 4

Carrot and Oats Pie

Each serving can be counted as three slices of light bread.

2 medium onions, chopped

3 tablespoons canola oil

6 medium carrots, coarsely grated

½ pound coarsely grated fresh pumpkin

1 cup 1%-fat milk

½ cup oats

⅓ cup raisins

Artificial sweetener (equivalent to 1 teaspoon sugar)

2 eggs, beaten

Salt, to taste

Preheat oven to 350°F.

In a large pot, sauté the onion in the oil until golden.

Add the carrots and pumpkin and continue sautéing, stirring continuously, for approximately 5 minutes.

Add the milk and bring to a boil. Lower the heat.

Add the oats and cook on low heat for approximately 3 minutes.

Add the remaining ingredients. Stir and cook for approximately 5 more minutes.

Transfer the mixture to a lightly greased pan (8" x 12" rectangular or 11" round) and bake for approximately 45 minutes until golden brown. Serve.

Serves 6 to 8

Buckwheat and Vegetable Casserole

Each serving can be counted as three slices of light bread.

¼ cup olive oil

1 large onion, finely diced

4 garlic cloves, crushed

2 red bell peppers, finely diced

1 carrot, coarsely grated

2 large tomatoes, diced

½ pound mushrooms, sliced

1 pound buckwheat

3 cups boiling water

1 tablespoon chicken-flavored instant bouillon

Salt and black pepper to taste

1 ounce chopped parsley, for garnish

In a large pan with a lid, heat the oil and add the onion, garlic, bell peppers, carrot, tomatoes, and mushrooms. Sauté for approximately 10 minutes until the vegetables are slightly soft.

Rinse the buckwheat in water (preferably boiling) and add to the pot to steam for a few more minutes.

Add the boiling water to the pot and season with the bouillon and salt and black pepper. Bring to a boil and lower the heat. Cover and cook for approximately 25 to 30 minutes.

Garnish with the parsley and serve.

Serves 6

Pearl Barley and Tomato Casserole

Each serving can be counted as two slices of light bread.

>
> 3 tablespoons olive or canola oil
>
> 1½ cups pearl barley
>
> 4 garlic cloves, sliced
>
> 1 pound tomatoes, chopped
>
> ½ pound mushrooms, sliced
>
> 2 ounces pitted black olives, sliced
>
> Salt and black pepper to taste
>
> 1 ounce chopped dill, for garnish

In a large pot, heat 2 tablespoons of the oil and fry the barley for a few minutes. Add water to cover barley by about 6 inches. Cover and cook for approximately 1 hour until the barley is soft. Drain and set aside.

In another large pot, heat the remaining tablespoon of oil and steam the garlic, tomatoes, mushrooms, and olives.

Add the barley and mix well.

Season with the salt and pepper. Garnish with the dill and serve.

Serves 6

Pepper and Cheese Pie

Each serving can be counted as two slices of light bread.

1 tablespoon canola oil

2 onions, chopped

1 pound mushrooms, sliced

1 pound feta cheese (5% fat)

3 eggs, beaten

2 tablespoons mushroom-flavored instant bouillon

1 tablespoon flour

Black pepper to taste

2 tablespoons fresh chopped dill, or 1 teaspoon dried

1 pickled red bell pepper, sliced

2 tablespoons breadcrumbs

Preheat oven to 350°F.

In a large frying pan, heat the oil and the onion and steam, covered, over a low flame until golden. If needed, add a teaspoon of water and continue steaming, stirring occasionally. Add the mushrooms and sauté, about 5 minutes. Remove from heat.

In a separate bowl, mix the cheese, eggs, instant bouillon, flour, pepper, and dill.

Lightly grease a heatproof 8" x 8" rectangular or 9" round and scatter the breadcrumbs on its bottom and along the sides. Add half of the cheese mixture and smooth the top. Pour the onion and mushroom on top and scatter the bell pepper slices. Top with the rest of the cheese mixture and smooth the top.

Bake in the preheated oven for approximately 40 minutes, until golden.

Serves 4-6

SOUPS AND SALADS ➤

Monks' Mixed Vegetable Bake

This casserole can be eaten in unlimited amounts.

1 large eggplant, cubed

1 large zucchini, cubed

2 medium carrots, chopped

4 medium onions, chopped

3 large bell peppers, chopped (use different colors, if desired)

1 cauliflower, chopped

½ pound green beans, cut

2 large ripe tomatoes, cubed

Sauce:

2 tablespoons olive oil

6 garlic cloves, crushed

1 can (4 ounces) tomato purée

1 teaspoon chicken-flavored instant bouillon

Salt and black pepper, to taste

Artificial sweetener to taste

Preheat the oven to 475°F.

Mix the vegetables together and scatter on the bottom of a lightly greased baking pan (8" x 12" rectangular or 11" round) and place in the oven. Bake for 20 minutes, stirring occasionally.

In the meantime, prepare the sauce. Add the olive oil to a large pot. Add the garlic, tomato purée, and bouillon. Stir.

Season the sauce with the salt and pepper and sweetener.

Cook the sauce on low heat for approximately 20 minutes. Add water as needed so the sauce does not become too thick.

Remove the vegetables from the oven when they are soft. Add them to the sauce. Stir gently and remove from heat. Serve.

Serves 8

Hummus and Rice Salad

Each serving can be counted as two pieces of light bread.

1 cup basmati rice

1 tablespoon canola oil

2 onions, diced

7 ounces canned hummus grains, without water

3 tablespoons chopped fresh chives

Salt and black pepper to taste

Make rice according to package directions. Remove from heat and cool, covered, until the rice reaches room temperature.

Heat the oil in a large frying pan, and then add the onion. Cover and steam over low heat until the onion is golden.

Transfer the rice to a bowl, add the hummus, onions, and chives, add salt and pepper to taste, and mix.

Serves 4

Minestrone Soup

This vegetable-based soup can be eaten in unlimited amounts.

½ cup white beans (or canned beans, drained)

1 medium onion, chopped

2 tablespoons olive or canola oil

2 carrots, diced

1 zucchini, diced

2 ripe tomatoes, chopped

2 cups water

1 cup tomato juice

1 tablespoon fresh basil, chopped

½ teaspoon fresh oregano, chopped

1 garlic clove, crushed

Salt and black pepper to taste

If you are using dried beans, soak them in water overnight. Discard the water, rinse the beans, and put in a heavy-bottomed pot. Add 1 quart of fresh water, or enough to cover the beans, and cook until the beans are soft. Drain and transfer the beans to a separate bowl.

In a large pot, sauté the onion in the oil until the onions are soft and translucent, about 10 minutes.

Add the carrot, and continue sautéing for about 10 minutes until they become soft. Add the zucchini and continue sautéing for 2 minutes. Add the tomatoes, water, tomato juice, herbs, and garlic and bring to a boil.

Lower the heat, season with salt and pepper, and cook for approximately 35 minutes. Add the cooked beans to the soup, simmer for 10 minutes, and serve.

Serves 6

Mushroom Soup

So easy to make! It can be eaten in unlimited amounts.

1 onion, sliced

1 pound mushrooms, sliced

2 garlic cloves, crushed

2 tablespoons canola oil

½ cup white wine

4 cups water

1 cup milk

5-6 stalks of thyme (optional)

2 tablespoons chicken-flavored instant bouillon

Salt and black pepper, to taste

Sauté the onion, mushrooms, and garlic in the oil.

Add the wine, water, and milk and bring to a boil. Add the thyme, if using.

Season with the bouillon and the salt and pepper.

Cook for 10 minutes and serve.

Serves 4

Mushroom and Yogurt Soup

One serving can be counted as half a portion of plain yogurt.

1 teaspoon canola oil

1 medium onion, sliced

2 garlic cloves, sliced

½ carrot, coarsely grated

1 celery stalk, finely chopped

1 pound mushrooms, sliced

2 cups water

2 stalks of thyme (optional)

1 tablespoon chicken-flavored instant bouillon

Salt and black pepper to taste

2 containers (6 ounces each) plain yogurt

In a deep pot, heat the oil and sauté the onion, garlic, carrot, celery, and mushrooms for approximately 15 minutes.

Add the water and thyme, if using, and bring to a boil.

Season with the bouillon and the salt and pepper and cook for approximately 5 more minutes.

Pour the yogurt into a large bowl, and gradually add 2 cups of the soup to the yogurt, stirring continuously. After the mixture is fully incorporated, return the mixture to the pot and stir.

Heat for a few more minutes, without bringing the soup to a boil, and serve.

Serves 4

Pumpkin Soup

This soup can be eaten in unlimited amounts.

> 1 tablespoon canola oil
>
> 1 teaspoon chopped ginger
>
> 1 large onion, finely chopped
>
> 1 medium carrot, chopped
>
> 2 celery stalks, chopped
>
> 2 pounds fresh pumpkin, diced
>
> 2 cups water
>
> 1 tablespoon chicken-flavored instant bouillon
>
> Salt and black pepper to taste
>
> Lemon juice to taste
>
> ½ teaspoon grated nutmeg

Heat the oil in a large heavy-bottomed pot and sauté the ginger.

Add the onion, carrot, celery, and pumpkin and sauté for approximately 20 minutes until all the vegetables are completely soft.

Add the water and the bouillon to the vegetables and bring to a boil.

Transfer to a food processor and process until smooth, about 1 minute, and season with the salt and pepper, lemon juice, and nutmeg. Serve.

Serves 6

Country-Style Bean Soup

One serving of this hearty soup can be counted as two slices of light bread.

⅓ pound white beans

⅓ pound chick-peas

1 medium onion, chopped

1 carrot, diced

2 garlic cloves, chopped

1 celeriac or celery stalk, chopped

1 red bell pepper, chopped

2 ripe tomatoes, diced

4 cups water

Salt and black pepper, to taste

2 tablespoons chicken-flavored instant bouillon

Soak the dried beans and chick-peas in water overnight. Pour off the water and add 1 quart of fresh water. Cook until the legumes are soft. Drain and set aside.

In a separate pot, steam the onion, carrot, garlic, celeriac, and bell pepper until the vegetables are soft.

Add the tomatoes and water to the vegetables.

Season with the salt and pepper and bouillon. Add the beans and chick-peas to the pot. Bring to a boil, then reduce the heat and simmer for 30 minutes.

Serves 6

Broccoli Soup

This dish can be eaten freely.

1 tablespoon canola oil

2 onions, diced

2 garlic cloves, sliced

1½ pounds fresh broccoli

2 zucchini, diced

4 tablespoons chicken-flavored instant bouillon

White pepper to taste

4 cups water

Heat the oil in a large pot and add the onion and garlic. Cover and steam over low flame until golden.

Add the broccoli, zucchini, instant bouillon, white pepper, and water. Stir.

Bring to a boil over a low flame until the vegetables are soft, about 15 minutes. Remove from heat.

Remove the broccoli stalks and separate the stalks from the flowers. Keep a few of the flowers aside for decoration. Chop the remaining broccoli and return to the pot and puree with a hand mixer. Pour into individual bowls and decorate each with the broccoli flowers.

Serves 4-6

EGGS ➤

Onion Quiche

One serving can be counted as two slices of light bread.

1 pound onions, sliced

1 tablespoon canola oil

1 pound leeks, trimmed and thinly sliced

1 bunch fresh chives, chopped

10 spring onions, chopped (use the whole onion)

3 bell peppers, finely diced (use different colors, if desired)

3 eggs, beaten

3 egg whites, beaten

4 garlic cloves, crushed

½ pound farmer cheese (up to 5% fat)

¼ cup breadcrumbs

½ cup parsley

1 teaspoon salt

¼ teaspoon black pepper

Nutmeg, to taste

Heat the oven to 325°F.

In a covered pot over low heat, sauté the onion in the oil until soft and golden.

Stir in the leeks, chives, and spring onions and continue sautéing for 5 to 7 more minutes.

Add the bell peppers and continue sautéing for 5 minutes.

Remove the pot from the heat. Set aside to cool and chill slightly.

Add the eggs, egg whites, garlic, cheese, breadcrumbs, parsley, and spices to the chilled mixture and stir.

Pour the mixture into a lightly greased pan (8" x 12" rectangular or 11" round) and bake for 45 minutes. Serve warm or at room temperature.

Serves 10

Spinach Quiche

Each serving can be counted as two slices of bread.

> 1 pound frozen spinach, thawed and drained
>
> 2 tablespoons potato flour
>
> 3 eggs, beaten
>
> 8-ounces 1%-fat milk
>
> ½ pound salted cheese (5% fat), crumbled
>
> 1 tablespoon olive oil
>
> 1 onion, chopped
>
> 1 tablespoon garlic clove, crushed
>
> Salt and black pepper to taste
>
> 2 tablespoons breadcrumbs

Preheat oven to 350°F.

In a bowl, combined the drained spinach, flour, eggs and milk. Add the cheese and mix.

Heat the oil in a large frying pan, add the onion, cover, and steam over low flame until golden. Add the steamed onion, garlic, salt, and pepper to the spinach bowl and mix.

Lightly grease a heatproof pan and scatter the breadcrumbs on its bottom and sides. Transfer the mixture to the pan. Bake in the preheated oven for approximately 40 minutes, until golden.

Serves 4-6

Zucchini, Tomato, and Tarragon Pie

One serving of pie can be counted as two slices of light bread.

2 medium onions, chopped

2 tablespoons olive oil

8 zucchini, thinly sliced

3 garlic cloves, crushed

½ pound cherry tomatoes, halved

2 tablespoons tarragon, coarsely chopped

1 bunch fresh chives, chopped

3 eggs, beaten

3 egg whites, beaten

1 teaspoon salt

¼ teaspoon black pepper

4 ounces low-fat ricotta

Preheat the oven to 350°F.

In a medium pot, sauté the onion in the oil until golden. Add the zucchini, garlic, tomatoes, tarragon, and chives and continue sautéing for 5 more minutes.

Add the eggs, egg whites, salt, and pepper and mix well.

Stir in the ricotta and mix well. Remove from the heat.

Pour the mixture into a lightly greased pan (8" x 12" rectangular or 11" round) and bake for approximately 45 minutes. Serve.

Serves 6

Egg and Broccoli Pie

Each serving can be counted as two slices of bread.

½ pound of cottage cheese (4% fat)

One 6-ounce container plain yogurt

3 eggs

2 tablespoons flour

2 tablespoons onion-flavored instant bouillon

White pepper to taste

2 pounds frozen broccoli, thawed and drained

2 slices low-fat hard cheese, such as cheddar (up to 9% fat)

Preheat oven to 350°F.

Mix the cottage cheese, yogurt, and eggs in a large bowl. Add the flour, instant bouillon, and white pepper, and stir. Add the broccoli and continue mixing until the broccoli is fully immersed.

Transfer to a lightly greased pan. Cut the hard cheese into narrow strips and put on top in crisscross fashion. Bake for approximately 40 minutes.

Serves 4-6.

Mushroom Pie

One serving can be counted as two slices of light bread.

1 onion, chopped

2 tablespoons canola oil

6 garlic cloves, crushed

2 pounds mushrooms, sliced (or canned mushrooms, drained)

Salt and black pepper to taste

2 tablespoons mushroom-flavored instant bouillon

¼ pound farmer cheese (up to 5% fat)

2 ounces low-fat cottage cheese

2 ounces low-fat feta cheese

6 egg whites (or 4 whole eggs)

Preheat the oven to 325°F.

In a large pot, sauté the onion in the oil. Add the garlic and mushrooms and continue sautéing for approximately 10 to 15 minutes.

Season with the salt and pepper and the bouillon.

Remove from the heat. Add the cheeses and let the mixture cool.

In a separate bowl, beat the egg whites (or the whole eggs) with a small amount of salt until stiff.

Gently fold the beaten egg whites (or the whole eggs) into the mushroom mixture.

Pour into a lightly greased pan (11" round) and bake for approximately 45 minutes. Serve hot.

Serves 6

Vegetable Omelet

This vegetable omelet can be eaten with two slices of light bread.

1 garlic clove, sliced

1 tablespoon olive oil

2-3 scallions, sliced

¼ cup grated carrot

4 Swiss chard leaves, sliced (without stems)

Salt and black pepper to taste

Lemon juice to taste

2 eggs + 2 egg whites, beaten

In a skillet, sauté the garlic in the oil.

Add the scallions, carrot, and Swiss chard, and continue cooking for a few more minutes.

Season with the salt, pepper, and lemon juice.

Pour the egg mixture over the vegetables. When the eggs are partially cooked, flip and continue cooking until the edges turn a golden brown.

Fry until golden brown on both sides. Serve.

Serves 2

Arugula and Herb Omelet

Arugula and Herb Omelet can be eaten with two slices of light bread.

2 eggs + 2 egg whites, beaten
¼ cup chopped arugula leaves
¼ cup chopped chives
¼ cup chopped parsley
Salt and black pepper to taste
1 teaspoon olive oil

In a small bowl, combine the egg mixture with the herbs and salt and pepper.

Heat the oil in a skillet. Pour the eggs into the skillet and fry until golden-brown on both sides.

Serves 2

Tomato and Onion Omelet

Tomato and Onion Omelet can be eaten with two slices of light bread.

1 large onion, chopped

1 tablespoon olive or canola oil

2 garlic cloves, crushed

1 small red bell pepper, diced

1 large ripe tomato, diced

Salt and black pepper to taste

Hot paprika to taste

2 eggs + 1 egg white, beaten

2 ounces feta cheese or goat cheese (up to 5% fat)

In a skillet, sauté the onion in the oil until golden.

Add the garlic, bell pepper, and tomato and continue sautéing for a few minutes.

Add the salt and pepper and paprika.

Add the eggs and cheese to the pan. When the underside of the omelet is ready, fold in half and serve.

Serves 2

Shakshuka (Israeli Omelet Dish)

Shakshuka can be eaten with two slices of light bread.

2 tablespoons olive oil

4 garlic cloves, chopped

1 red bell pepper, diced

2 large ripe tomatoes, diced

2-3 tablespoons tomato purée

Artificial sweetener (equivalent to 1 teaspoon sugar)

Salt and black pepper to taste

¼ teaspoon hot paprika (optional)

1 tablespoon sweet paprika

¼ ounce coriander or parsley, chopped

3 whole eggs

Slightly heat the oil in a deep frying pan over medium heat. Add the garlic and sauté until golden.

Stirring constantly, add the following ingredients, waiting a few minutes between each: bell pepper, tomato, tomato purée, artificial sweetener, salt, hot paprika (if using), and sweet paprika.

Last, add the coriander or parsley and lower the heat.

Make a few depressions in the mixture. Crack the eggs and put one in each depression. Be careful not to break the yolk. Cover and cook on low heat for a few minutes until the eggs are set. Serve.

Serves 2

Mushroom and Onion Omelet

Mushroom and Onion Omelet can be eaten with two slices of light bread.

1 small onion, diced

1 tablespoon olive or canola oil

1 garlic clove, crushed

½ pound mushrooms, sliced

Salt and black pepper to taste

Nutmeg to taste (optional)

1 bunch fresh chives, coarsely chopped

2 eggs + 1 egg white, beaten

In a skillet, sauté the onion in the oil until golden. Add the garlic and mushrooms and continue sautéing.

Season with the salt and pepper and the nutmeg, if using. Add the chives.

Pour the egg mixture into the pan.

Fry for a few minutes, turn over, and serve.

Serves 2

SAUCES & DRESSINGS ➤

Balsamic Vinaigrette

This salad dressing can be added to foods freely.

½ tablespoon Dijon mustard

3 garlic cloves, crushed

5 tablespoons olive oil

¼ cup balsamic vinegar

1 tablespoon freshly squeezed lemon juice

2-3 thyme leaves, minced

Salt and black pepper, to taste

Pinch of artificial sweetener

Combine the mustard and garlic in a small bowl. Whisk in the oil.

Whisk in the vinegar, lemon juice, and thyme. Season with the salt and pepper and sweetener.

Put in a glass jar with a tight lid. Keep refrigerated. Shake each time before use.

Makes approximately 1 cup

Napolitana Sauce for Pasta

This sauce can be added to foods freely.

> 3 large garlic cloves, crushed
>
> 1-2 tablespoons olive oil
>
> 5 large ripe tomatoes, chopped
>
> 1 can (4 ounces) tomato purée
>
> Salt to taste
>
> 5-6 fresh basil leaves
>
> Artificial sweetener to taste

In a medium pot, sauté the garlic in the olive oil.

Stir in the tomatoes and tomato purée. Cook for approximately 20 minutes.

Add the salt, basil, and artificial sweetener to the sauce, until the desired flavor is obtained.

Makes 4 to 6 servings

Yogurt Sauce

One to two tablespoons makes an excellent topping for pasta.

1 container (6 ounces) plain yogurt

2 tablespoons Dijon mustard

3 tablespoons finely crushed garlic cloves

3 tablespoons olive oil

1 teaspoon mustard seeds (optional)

1 tablespoon chopped chives

Salt and black pepper to taste

Mix all the ingredients in a small bowl. Cover and refrigerate for 2 to 3 hours before using. The sauce will keep for about 1 week.

Makes approximately 1 cup

BIBLIOGRAPHY

Blum, I.; L. Nessiel; E. Graff; A. Harsat; O Raz, and Y. Vered. "Food Preferences, Body Weight and Platelet Poor Plasma (PPP) Serotonin, and Catecholamines," *American Journal of Clinical Nutrition,* 57 (1993): 486–89.

Blum, I.; Y. Vered; E. Graff; Y. Groskopf; A. Harsat; and O. Raz. "The Influence of Meal Composition on Plasma Serotonin and Norepinephrine," *Metabolism,* 41 (1992): 137–40.

Brand Miller, J.; K. Foster-Powel; and S. Colagiuri. *The G.I. Factor: The Glycemic Index Solution* (Sydney: Hodder Headline, 1996).

Bray, G. A. "Progress in Understanding the Genetics of Obesity," *The Journal of Nutrition,* Vol. 127, No. 5 (May 1997): 940S–942S.

Bray, G. A. "Genetic, Hypothalamic and Endocrine Features of Clinical and Experimental Obesity," *Progress in Brain Research,* 93 (1992): 333–41.

Brown, Judith E. *Nutrition Now,* 2d ed. (Belmont, Calif.: Wadsworth Publishing Company, 1999).

Buchhorn, D. "Adjusted Carbohydrate Exchange: Food Exchanges for Diabetes Management Corrected with the Glycemic Index," *Australian Journal of Nutrition and Dietetics,* 54 (1997): 55–68.

Carey, V. J., et al. "Body Fat Distribution and Risk of NIDDM in Women," *American Journal of Epidemiology* 145 (1997): 614–19.

Chahad, G.; Y. W. Ande; and J. L. Mehta. "Dietary Recommendations in the Prevention and Treatment of Coronary Heart Disease: Do We Have the Ideal Diet Yet?" *American Journal of Cardiology,* 94 (2004): 1260–67.

"Clinical guidelines on the identification, evaluation and treatment of overweight and obesity in adults," *National Institutes of Health,* NIH publication No. 98-4083 (1998).

Colditz, G. A. "Economic Costs of Obesity," *American Journal of Clinical Nutrition,* 55 (1992): 503S–507S.

Dandona, P.; A. Aljada; A. Chaudhuri; P. Mohanty; and R. Garg. "Metabolic Syndrome: A Comprehensive Perspective Based on Interaction between Obesity, Diabetes and Inflammation," *Circulation,* Vol. 111, No. 11 (March 22, 2005): 1448–54.

Dansinger, M. L., et. al. "Composition of the Atkins, Ornish, Weight Watchers, and Zone Diets for Weight Loss and Heart Disease Risk Reduction," *The Journal of the American Medical Association,* 293:1 (2005): 43–53.

De Castro, J. "Eating Behavior: Lessons from the Real World of Humans," *Nutrition,* 16 (2000): 800–813.

Eckel, R. H. "The Dietary Approach to Obesity," *The Journal of the American Medical Association,* 293:1 (2005): 96–97.

Guy-Grand, B., and G. Ailhaud, eds. *Progress in Obesity Research.* 8th International Congress of Obesity (London: John Libbey, 1999).

Holt, S. H. A.; J. C. Brand Miller; and P. Petocz. "An Insulin Index of Foods: The Insulin Demand Generated by 1000-kJ Portions of Common Foods," *American Journal of Clinical Nutrition,* 66 (1997): 1264–76.

Jenkins, D. J. A., et al. "Starchy Food and Glycemic Index," *Diabetes Care,* 11 (1988): 149–59.

Kalergis, M., et al. "Attempts to Control the Glycemic Response to Carbohydrates in Diabetes Mellitus: Overview and Practical Implications," *Canadian Journal of Diabetes Care,* 22 (1998): 20–29.

Karanja, N. M. "Descriptive Characteristics of the Dietary Approach to Stop Hypertension Trial," *Journal of American Dietetic Association,* 99 (1999): S19-S27.

Lemonick, M.D. "The Mood Molecule," *Time,* 15 (1997): 74–83.

Levin, B. E., and V. H. Routh. "Role of the Brain in Energy Balance and Obesity," *American Journal of Physiology,* 27 (1996): R491–R500.

Ludwig, D. S., et al. "High Glycemic Index Foods, Overeating and Obesity," *Pediatrics,* 103 (1999): e26–32.

McLaughlin, T.; F. Abbasi; K. Cheal; J Chu; C. Lamendola; and G. Reaven. "Use of Metabolic Markers to Identify Overweight Individuals Who Are Insulin Resistant," *Annals of Internal Medicine,* Vol. 139, No. 10 (November 18, 2003): 802–9.

Meguid, M., et al. "Hypothalamic Dopamine and Serotonin in the Regulation of Food Intake," *Nutrition,* 16 (2000): 843–57.

Monro, J. A. "Glycaemic Glucose Equivalent: Combining Carbohydrate Content, Quantity and Glycaemic Index of Foods for Precision in Gycemia Management," *Asia Pacific Journal of Clinical Nutrition,* Vol. 11, No. 3 (September 2002): 217–25.

Pi-Sunyer, F. X. "Energy Balance: Role of Genetics and Activity," *New York Academy of Science*, Vol. 819, No. 1 (May 23, 1997): 29–36.

"Point/Counterpoint Glycemic Index: Pro and Con," *Nutrition Today*, 34 (March/April 1999): 64–88. A series of articles on the advantages and disadvantages of the glycemic index by experts in the field, including Janette Brand-Miller and Kaye Foster-Powell, Thomas M. S. Wolever (pro), Marion J. Franz, Christine Beebe (con), and Helen Katanas (pro).

Reaven, G. M. "Role of Insulin Resistance in Human Disease," *Diabetes*, 37 (1988): 1595–1607.

Reaven, G.; F. Abbasi; and T. McLaughlin. "Obesity, Insulin Resistance, and Cardiovascular Disease," *Recent Progress in Hormone Research*, 59 (January 1, 2004): 207–23.

Rosenbaum, M., et al. "Obesity," *New England Journal of Medicine*, 337 (1997): 396–407.

Salmeron, J., et al. "Dietary Fiber, Glycemic Load and Risk of NIDDM in Men," *Diabetes Care*, 2 (1997): 545–50.

Salmeron, J., et al. "Dietary Fiber, Glycemic Load and Risk of NIDDM in Women," *The Journal of the American Medical Association*, 12 (1997): 472–77.

Sheard, N. D., N. G. Clare, et al. "Dietary Carbohydrates (Amount and Type) in the Prevention of Diabetes," *Diabetes Care*, Vol. 27, No. 9 (September 2004): 2266–71.

Shils, M. E.; J. A. Olson; M. Shike; and A. C. Poss. *Modern Nutrition in Health and Disease*, 9th ed. (Philadelphia, Pa.: Lippincott Williams & Wilkins, 1999).

Whitney, E. N., and S. R. Rolfes. *Understanding Nutrition*, 10th ed. (Belmont, Calif.: Wadsworth Publishing Company, 2004).

Willet, W.; J. Manson; and S. Lau. "Glycemic Index, Glycemic Load, and Risk of Type 2 Diabetes," *American Journal of Clinical Nutrition*, Vol. 76, No. 1 suppl. (July 1, 2002): S274–80.

Wolf, A., and G. Colditz. "Current Estimates of the Economic Cost of Obesity in the United States," *Obesity Research*, 6 (1998): 97.

INDEX

A

acupuncture, 170

alcohol, 100–101, 113, 182; calories in, 101, 113; gender and, 101, 113

American Diabetes Association, 89

anorexia, 165

antidepressants, 48, 67, 70, 119

antioxidants, 85, 100

appetite, 40, 54, 153, 156, 170

arteriosclerosis, 166

Arugula and Herb Omelet, 218

B

Balsamic Vinaigrette, 224

Barley and Vegetable Casserole, 194

Beet Leaf and Chick-Pea Casserole, 195

Blood Brain Barrier (BBB), 43, 44, 45

blood sugar. *see also* glucose: abdominal obesity and, 25; Bread for Life Diet and, 76; diabetes and, 69, 79; exercise and, 75, 154; high-protein diet and, 165; hypoglycemia and, 69; insulin and, 52; satiety and, 30; skipping meals and, 74; vegetables and, 85

body fat, 149; abdominal, 25, 26, 55, 76; age and, 23; Bread for Life Diet and, 65; burning, 75; calories and, 148; glycemic index and, 59, 104; insulinemia and, 54; obesity and, 24; percentage, 24, 27, 164; triclycerides and, 70; weight gain and, 118–19, 164

Body Mass Index (BMI), 21, 22, 27, 122, 171; calculating, 21

bone density, 154

brain: carbohydrates and, 183; hunger and, 34; hunger-satiety center and, 40; neurotransmitters and, 13; sensory perception and, 33–34; serotonin and, 43; weight and, 28–30, 129–30

bread: calories and, 13; celiac disease and, 178; combination diets and, 167; daily eating plan and, 80; daily portion, 14; diabetes and, 68; diets and, 72; glycemic index and, 64; light, 13, 78, 80, 81, 102, 112; meat meal and, 91, 93; satiety and, 13; serotonin and, 13, 46, 64; Stage I and, 77, 104, 107; Stage II and, 108; substitutes, 68, 77, 81, 108, 109–11; types of, 81, 82; weight loss and, 183; white, 13, 78, 81, 176; whole grain, 80, 176

Bread for Life Diet; approach of, 12; benefits of, 65, 70, 76, 141; blood pressure and, 68, 184; blood sugar and, 76; the brain and, 40; cholesterol and, 184; cravings and, 51; depression and, 48; diabetics and, 180, 184; eating and, 33, 134–35, 172; eating plan, 80; exercise and, 157, 185; family and, 124; FAQs about, 173–85; health and, 66, 70–71; insulin and, 53, 56, 65; metabolism and, 164; mood and, 50; principles of, 12, 67, 73, 74–76, 104, 108, 174; recipes, 80, 187, 189–221; sample day, 80, 106, 114–17; serotonin and, 29, 41, 50, 71; Stage I, 77, 78–79, 80, 91, 96, 103–7, 111, 117; Stage II, 77, 79–80, 96, 101, 102, 109–17, 175; weight loss and, 13, 50

bread portions: for men, 80, 91, 102, 104, 105, 108, 111; for women, 80, 91, 102,

104, 105, 111, 198

Broccoli Soup, 209

Buckwheat and Vegetable Casserole, 197

butter, 83, 94, 95, 97, 165

C

caffeine, 99–100

calcium, 102, 103, 105, 107, 112

calories, 150; alcohol and, 101, 113; bread
    and, 80; burning, 146, 150, 152, 153,
    154; counting, 72, 73, 104, 144, 147, 177;
    energy and, 144; metabolism and, 163,
    180; nutrients and, 148; sweets and, 46;
    vegetables and, 85; yo-yo dieting and,
    164

cancer, 85, 100, 101, 150

carbohydrates, 66, 75; blood sugar and,
    57, 64; function of, 165; glycemic index
    and, 59, 61 (chart); hunger and, 43;
    meat meal and, 91, 93; restrictive diets
    and, 166; serotonin and, 43, 45, 46;
    weight loss and, 183

carbohydrates, complex, 147, 148, 149
    (listed); Bread for Life Diet and, 74, 108,
    150; diabetes and, 79, 180; health bene-
    fits of, 68–71; modern diet and, 122;
    serotonin and, 46, 48, 144

carbohydrates, simple, 148, 149 (listed);
    insulin level and, 56, 74; serotonin and,
    46, 48

Carrot and Oats Pie, 196

celiac disease, 68, 178

cephalic phase, 36, 37, 39, 75

cereal, breakfast, 110–11

cheese, 83, 84, 95, 112, 165

Chinese Vegetable Stir-Fry, 193

cholesterol: animal fat and, 91, 149; Atkins
    diet and, 166; Bread for Life Diet and,
    15, 65, 67, 68, 69–70, 76, 184; cooking

oils and, 95; exercise and, 154; fats and,
    96; metabolic syndrome and, 54; obesity
    and, 26

coffee, 95, 99–100

concentration, impaired, 76, 166

constipation, 67, 70–71

cooking methods, 58, 85, 88, 93, 95

corn, 85, 86, 91, 104, 149; as bread substi-
    tute, 87, 110, 178

cortisol, 26

cortisone, 119

Country-Style Bean Soup, 208

cravings, 13, 70, 132; Bread for Life Diet
    and, 49, 134; calories and, 73; complex
    carbohydrates and, 49; diabetes and, 69;
    habits and, 138; high-protein diets and,
    45, 47, 165; hyperinsulinemia and, 54,
    58; serotonin and, 42, 43, 50, 51, 60

C-Reactive Protein (CRP), 68

D

dairy products, 67, 80, 94–95, 112, 149,
    165

dehydration, 70, 75, 79, 99, 165, 166

depression: Bread for Life Diet and, 48;
    eating and, 126; protein and, 45, 60;
    serotonin and, 41, 42, 48

diabetes: Bread for Life Diet and, 65, 66,
    67, 68–69, 79; environment and, 121;
    hyperinsulinemia and, 58; obesity and,
    54; syndrome X and, 26

diet, 35, 72, 150; Atkins, 166; blood type,
    168; carbohydrate-restricted, 165, 166;
    combination, 167–68; crash, 145, 147,
    150; high-protein, 46, 48, 165, 166; juice,
    168–69; liquid, 168; low-calorie, 145,
    150, 163, 164–65; mono, 167–68; pills,
    170; Scarsdale, 166; South Beach, 166;
    Weight Watchers, 169; Zone, 166

dieting, 161; action plan for, 136–41;
Bread for Life Diet and, 12; eating problems and, 127–35; health problems and,
168–69; myths about, 172–85; rigid
approach to, 72, 127; succeeding at,
129–30; teenage girls and, 161, 162;
women and, 163, 166; yo-yo, 24, 163, 164
diuretics, 170

E

eating: cephalic phase of, 36, 37, 39, 75;
enjoyment of, 129–30, 134; between
meals, 177; at night, 98, 104, 132, 178;
reasons for, 31, 126–27; the senses and,
34; slowly, 138; uncontrolled, 177; while
cooking, 103; while distracted, 130–31,
134, 181
eating behavior, 38, 47, 123, 133; changing, 37, 119, 126–41; conditioned, 35,
36, 132, 138, 183; destructive, 127–35;
habits, 36, 78, 130, 132, 139, 141, 174;
neuropeptides and, 30; relationships
and, 139–40; weight gain and, 119
Egg and Broccoli Pie, 215
eggs, 94–95, 104, 112, 163
endorphins, 153, 156
energy, 146–147, 166; balance, 73, 143–50
exercise, 55, 75, 120, 146, 151–60, 180,
184–85; gender and, 153; heart disease
and, 153; weight-bearing, 154, 156

F

fasting, 145, 147, 171
fats, 96, 121, 144, 148, 149, 183; animal,
149; hydrogenated, 97, 150; monounsaturated, 95, 150; saturated, 69, 83, 95,
166; unsaturated, 94; vegetable, 69, 149
fiber: benefits of, 69, 70–71; breakfast
cereal and, 110; carbohydrates and, 148;

fruit and, 89; glycemic index and, 149;
modern diet and, 122; vegetables and,
85, 88
fish, 84, 91–94, 105; heart disease and, 93
fluids, 70–71, 75, 107; gender and, 78, 79,
99, 105, 195
food: declining, 133, 181; deprivation,
134, 136, 137; diary, 130–31, 175–76;
energy, 143, 144; limited, recommended,
77, 78; shopping, 39, 40, 123, 134, 138,
179–80; simple, 31, 33; unlimited, recommended, 77, 78, 86 (listed), 104
frame size, 19, 20, 23
fruit, 89–91; blood sugar and, 79; Bread
for Life Diet and, 77; calories, 182; craving for sweets and, 132; fructose and, 89,
149; glycemic index and, 64; juice, 91,
169; meat meal and, 138; serving size,
90; in Stage I, 107; in Stage II, 104, 112

G

gastric surgery, 171
glucose, 52, 57, 64, 68, 69, 148, 165; tolerance test, 58
glycemic index, 57, 60; Bread for Life Diet
and, 73; carbohydrates and, 61 (chart),
74, 144; factors affecting, 59; food chart
and, 62–63; fruit and, 91, 104, 112;
glucose-based, 57; grains and, 109; vegetables and, 85; white-bread-based, 57,
62–63; whole grain bread and, 81
glycogen, 148
Green Fettuccine with Roasted Vegetables,
190

H

headaches, 43, 70, 170
heartburn (acid reflux), 67, 71
heart disease, 68; animal fat and, 149;

Bread for Life Diet and, 65, 66, 67; exercise and, 153, 159; fish and, 93; hyperinsulinemia and, 54; obesity and, 25; syndrome X and, 25; tea and, 100

high blood pressure (hypertension): Bread for Life Diet and, 65, 67, 184; diabetes and, 54; exercise and, 154; obesity and, 26; omega 3 fatty acids and, 93

Hummus and Rice Salad, 203

hunger: the brain and, 28, 40; Bread for Life Diet and, 12, 40, 104, 136, 172; carbohydrates and, 43, 49; eating frequently and, 77, 98; food shopping and, 179; high-protein diets and, 165; hunger center and, 39; minimizing, 103, 134; portion size and, 39; satiety and, 29–32, 40; serotonin and, 13, 73; skipping meals and, 70, 74, 98; social events and, 131; sweets and, 45–47; weight loss and, 56

hyperinsulinemia, 25, 53, 54, 55, 58, 68

hypoglycemia, 26, 58, 67

hypothalamus, 29, 40

hypothyroidism, 119

I

inflammation, 15, 26, 55, 93

insulin: big meals and, 94; Bread for Life Diet and, 15, 76; carbohydrates and, 74, 82, 144; diabetes and, 68–69, 180; eating frequently and, 97; excess, 53; physical activity and, 154; small meals and, 75; Stage II and, 79; tryptophan and, 45; vegetables and, 85; weight gain and, 52–65, 73

insulin resistance: Bread for Life Diet and, 15, 56; hyperinsulinemia and, 53, 58; serotonin and, 54

L

laxatives: weight loss and, 170; women and, 170

legumes, 85, 87, 108–9, 149; as bread substitute, 87, 108

liposuction, 172

liver, 148

M

margarine, 83, 94, 96, 150

meals: Bread for Life Diet and, 77; meat, 91, 93, 102, 105, 107, 111; sample, 80

meals, frequent: Bread for Life Diet and, 77, 80, 97–98, 104; diabetes and, 79; health and, 68–71; insulin and, 56; sample day and, 106; serotonin and, 48, 74; weight loss and, 50

meals, skipping: blood sugar and, 74, 79; Bread for Life Diet and, 102, 134; excess eating and, 181; headaches and, 70; hunger and, 98, 134; metabolism and, 145; serotonin and, 74

meals, small: benefits of, 49, 75; Bread for Life Diet and, 79; health issues and, 68–71; protein and, 94

meat, 75; adolescents and, 67; Bread for Life Diet and, 77, 80, 91–94, 105, 111; children and, 67; combination diets and, 167; cooking methods, 95; high-protein diets and, 165; pregnancy and, 67

medications, 119, 170, 196

menopause, 23

metabolism, 75, 98, 143, 152, 163, 164, 180; age and, 145; basal, 143–45, 147, 152; gender and, 145; problems with, 119; smoking and, 146

milk, 94–95, 99, 100, 149, 167

Minestrone Soup, 204

Monks' Mixed Vegetable Bake, 202

monosodium glutamate (MSG), 75

mood, 76; Bread for Life Diet and, 50; high-protein diets and, 165; serotonin and, 43, 60, 64, 70, 71, 73, 74

muscles, 145, 146, 152, 164, 165, 171, 184

Mushroom and Onion Omelet, 221

Mushroom and Yogurt Soup, 206

Mushroom Pie, 216

Mushroom Soup, 205

N

Napolitana Sauce for Pasta, 225

neurotransmitters, 13, 40, 70

nutrients, 73, 78, 94; color and, 85–86; labels and, 82, 97, 111; types of, 148

O

obesity, 16–17; animals and, 30; apple-shaped (abdominal), 25, 26, 55; Body Mass Index (BMI) and, 21, 171; child-hood, 121, 123, 124; culture and, 16; diabetes and, 54; diet-induced, 162; epidemic, 118, 122; gender and, 122; heredity and, 119–25, 121, 136, 146, 151, 180; hyperinsulinemia and, 53, 54; mor-bid, 171; pear-shaped, 25; Pima Indians and, 121–22; psychology and, 16, 47; research, 14–15, 31, 41, 53, 121, 134, 163; self-image and, 16; types of, 25, 26; women and, 16

oil, vegetable: Bread for Life Diet and, 95; cholesterol and, 69, 94; cooking meth-ods and, 87, 96; daily portion of, 95, 105, 107, 113; high blood pressure and, 68; recommended types, 150

olives, 96

omega 3 fatty acids, 93

Onion Quiche, 212

osteoporosis, 154

overeating, 36, 39, 78, 131, 132, 174; rationalizations for, 135, 150

overweight: Body Mass Index (BMI) and, 21, 122; Bread for Life Diet and, 66; chil-dren, 123; defining, 18; exercise and, 135; habits and, 78; insulin levels and, 53; population, 122; running and, 159; self-acceptance and, 128

P

pasta, 109, 149

Pasta and Sun-Dried-Tomato Salad, 191

Pearl Barley and Tomato Casserole, 198

Pepper and Cheese Pie, 199

physical activity. see also exercise: aerobic, 152; anaerobic, 153; Bread for Life Diet and, 73, 75; calorie burning, 75, 146, 152, 154, 155 (listed); children and, 123; energy balance and, 142–43; exercise, 151–60; fat and, 24; hunger and, 132, 139; obesity epidemic and, 118; partner and, 140; weight gain and, 18, 121, 122; work and, 120

phytochemicals, 86, 88, 89

PMS, 67, 70

polyphenols, 100

portion size, 38–39, 40, 152

potatoes, 86, 91, 104, 149; as bread substi-tute, 87, 110; protein and, 167; starch content and, 85

poultry, 91–94, 95, 111

prediabetes, 55, 69, 78

pregnancy, 67, 120

protein: blood sugar and, 59; Bread for Life Diet and, 12, 91–94, 183; calories and, 144; energy and, 147; function of, 148; legumes and, 108; low-carbohydrate diets and, 165–67; preference for, 50;

serotonin and, 13, 59, 64

Pumpkin Soup, 207

R

recipes, 189–226

restaurants: Bread for Life Diet and, 73, 104; challenges of, 32; choosing, 138; meat meal and, 93, 105; ordering in, 102, 178; portion size in, 38

rice, 109, 149, 178

Rice Salad, 192

S

sandwiches, 77, 78, 103, 139; spreads for, 83, 84, 104

satiety: the brain and, 28; Bread for Life Diet and, 75; cephalic phase and, 36; hunger and, 31; hypothalamus and, 29, 30; satiety center and, 30; serotonin and, 13, 49; vegetables and, 85

seafood, 93

Seasonal Affective Disorder (SAD), 42, 43

self-image, 76, 128–29, 139

serotonin, 70; appetite and, 54; bread and, 13, 64, 82; Bread for Life Diet and, 29; carbohydrates and, 42, 43, 46, 48, 71; cravings and, 132; depression and, 43, 45, 60; diet pills and, 170; eating frequently and, 97; food and, 13; gender and, 44, 45, 50, 165; hunger and, 13, 29, 40, 46, 47, 73, 132; neurotransmitters and, 13; obesity and, 42; protein and, 13, 43, 45, 60, 132; research and, 13, 41–51; satiety and, 13, 29, 40; sleep and, 99; small meals and, 75; snacks and, 111; social factors and, 44; sweets and, 165; weight loss and, 41–51

Shakshuka (Israeli Omelet Dish), 220

sleep apnea, 99

smoking, 146

snoring, 99

social events: Bread for Life Diet and, 73; challenges of, 32, 129, 133, 176, 177; hunger and, 131

soy products, 92, 95, 112

spas, weight loss, 171

Spinach Quiche, 213

starch, 18, 87, 108, 149

starvation, 49

steroids, 119

stress, 58, 71, 120; hormones, 55, 58, 145

stroke, 54

sugar, 64–65; alcohol and, 113; artificial sweeteners and, 100; breakfast cereal and, 110; fluids and, 99, 169, 182; fruit and, 91, 95; fruit juice and, 169; nutrition labels and, 82; simple carbohydrates and, 148; triglycerides and, 70

sweeteners, artificial, 95, 99, 100, 112

sweet potatoes, 85, 86, 91, 104; as bread substitute, 87, 110

sweets, 50, 132; avoiding, 69, 77; Bread for Life Diet and, 112–13; children and, 123, 124; excuses and, 135; gastric surgery and, 171; guilt and, 47, 84, 128, 133; overeating and, 174; snacks and, 183; temptation and, 139

syndrome X (metabolic syndrome), 25, 26, 54, 55

T

taste, sense of, 33, 34, 129–30

tea, 99–100

thyroid, 145

Tomato and Onion Omelet, 219

trans-fatty acids, 96, 97, 150

triglycerides: abdominal obesity and, 26; Bread for Life Diet and, 15, 67, 70, 76;

exercise and, 184; heart disease and, 68; syndrome X and, 54

tryptophan, 43, 44, 45

U

uric acid, 165

V

Vegetable Omelet, 217

vegetables, 85–89; benefits of, 69–70; Bread for Life Diet and, 77; fruit and, 90, 114; goals and, 138; meat meal and, 91; salads and, 95; sandwiches and, 78, 103; Stage I and, 80; Stage II and, 80, 104, 105, 111

vegetarians, 92, 94

vitamins and minerals: Bread for Life Diet and, 74; combination diets and, 167; complex carbohydrates and, 69; fruit and, 89; nutrient groups and, 148; protein and, 91; supplements, 75, 102, 105, 107; vegetables and, 85, 86, 87–88

W

waist measurement, 27; gender and, 26, 27; obesity type and, 25, 26, 55

water, 70, 75, 132, 148, 182

weight, 20; age and, 18, 22, 23; gender and, 18, 20, 22, 23, 119–20; optimal, 19, 20, 23

weight gain: after diet, 160, 162; age and, 185; basal metabolism and, 143; behavior and, 36, 119; biology of, 118; Bread for Life Diet and, 73; calories and, 144; causes of, 23, 31, 119, 122; eating at night and, 178; energy balance and, 142; environment and, 119–25, 139; gastric surgery and, 171; gender and, 119, 185; heredity and, 119, 120–22, 123, 125, 128,

146; insulin and, 65; lifestyle and, 122–23, 124; skipping meals and, 98; yo-yo dieting and, 163

weight loss: abdominal obesity and, 26; action plan, 135–41; attitudes and, 76, 126–41, 147; basal metabolism and, 143; behavior and, 126–41; bread and, 183; Bread for Life Diet and, 13, 15, 66, 76, 160, 172; combination diets and, 167; commitment and, 136–37; crash diets and, 145; dehydration and, 98; energy balance and, 142; exercise and, 152; factors influencing, 60; fasting and, 171; goals, 27, 129, 136, 137–39, 140, 162; gradual, 27, 137, 185; high-protein diets and, 165; hunger-satiety and, 30; insulin and, 54, 56; juice diets and, 169; laxatives and, 170; methods, 169–72; mono diets and, 166; obstacles and, 130–34; partnerships and, 139–40, 141; plateau, 164; serotonin and, 41–51; speed of, 185; Stage I and, 103; succeeding at, 173–85; walking and, 156; yo-yo dieting and, 162, 163

Weight Watchers, 169

women, 18, 20, 23; exercise and, 153; high-protein diets and, 46; laxatives and, 170

X

Xenical, 171

Y

yogurt, 95, 102

Yogurt Sauce, 226

Z

Zucchini, Tomato, and Tarragon Pie, 214

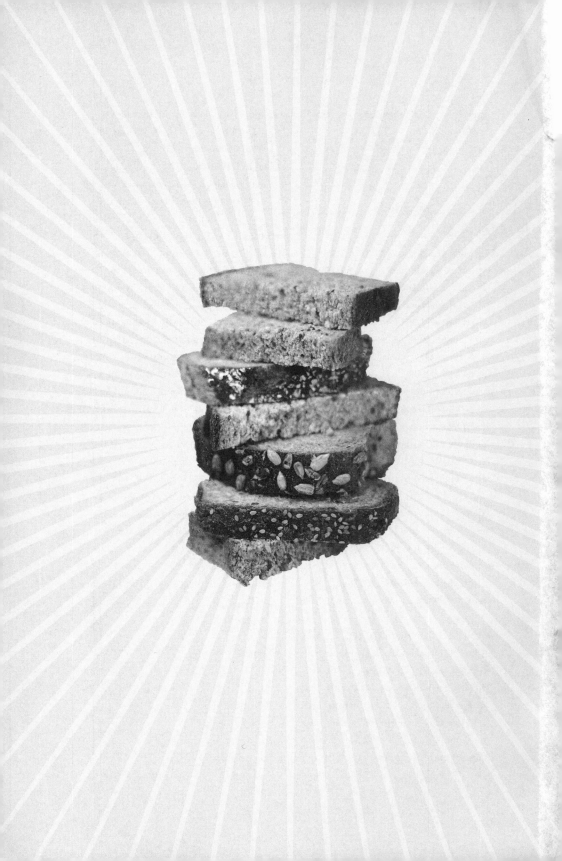